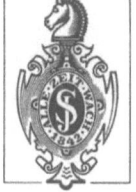

D. Ottoson   T. Lundeberg

# Pain Treatment by
# TENS Transcutaneous Electrical Nerve
A Practical Manual Stimulation

With 79 Figures

Springer-Verlag
Berlin Heidelberg New York
London Paris Tokyo

Prof. Davɪᴅ Oᴛᴛᴏsᴏɴ

Associate Prof. Tʜᴏᴍᴀs Lᴜɴᴅᴇʙᴇʀɢ

Department of Physiology II
Karolinska Institutet

S-10401 Stockholm

ISBN-13: 978-3-540-19206-0      e-ISBN-13: 978-3-642-73624-7

DOI: 10.1007/ 978-3-642-73624-7

Library of Congress Cataloging-in-Publication Data. Ottoson, David, 1918–   TENS: transcutaneous electrical nerve stimulation/D. Ottoson, T. Lundeberg. p.   cm.   Bibliography: p.   Includes index.

1. Transcutaneous electrical nerve stimulation. I. Lundeberg, T. (Thomas), 1953–   . II. Title. RM880.O88 1988   616'.0472–dc19

© Springer-Verlag Berlin Heidelberg 1988
© Illustrations: David Ottoson and Thomas Lundeberg
**Softcover reprint of the hardcover 1st edition 1988**

Reproduction of figures: Gustav Dreher GmbH, Stuttgart

Typesetting, printing, and bookbinding: Petersche Druckerei GmbH & Co. Offset KG, Rothenburg ob der Tauber

2125/3130-543210 – Printed on acid-free paper

# Preface

The relief of pain is one of the most important problems in medicine. For centuries various forms of analgesic drugs were the only means by which pain could be combatted. Recent decades have witnessed a dramatic progress in pain research which has provided new insights into the neurophysiological basis of pain. The discoveries of the physiological mechanisms of pain control have led to new conceptual aspects of the perception of pain. Even more important is that these discoveries have paved the way for the development of new techniques and methods for the alleviation of pain.

One of these methods is transcutaneous electrical nerve stimulation (TENS). This method emerged from the concept of the gate control theory which was proposed by Melzack and Wall in 1965 and introduced into clinical practice in 1970. In the years which have passed since then, TENS has become widely used, and there is at present abundant evidence that it provides an efficient tool for the alleviation of certain pain syndromes. In spite of the increasing use of TENS, there is no short practical manual for its application. The present book tries to fill this gap and also provides a brief introduction to the neurophysiological basis of pain and the pain-relieving effects of TENS.

D. OTTOSON
T. LUNDEBERG

# Contents

*Chapter 3*
TENS in Different Pain Syndromes

*Chapter 4*
Additional Areas of Application of TENS and Different Modes
of Electrical Stimulation

# *Chapter 1*   The Neurophysiology of Pain

Pain arises as a result of signals in specific nerves that travel to the brain. In describing the neurophysiological processes of pain it is usual to proceed from the receptors which generate the pain signals in the pain nerves to the transmission processes at various levels of the routes to the final end station in the brain. There follows a brief outline of the anatomy of the afferent pain system and the main steps in the neurophysiological processes underlying the generation and transmission of pain signals.

Pain Receptors

Sensory nerves form, in the skin and other tissues, a variety of sensory endings or receptors, such as Meissner's and Pacini's corpuscles, Krause's bulbs, Ruffini's endings, etc. In addition to these endings, which are all encapsulated, there are also free naked nerve endings which form bushy networks of thin nerve fibres (see Fig. 1.1). It is generally agreed that some of these nerve endings represent the specific pain receptors. They are found in almost all tissues but the density of fibres differs greatly from one organ to another. Thus highly pain-sensitive tissues such as the cornea and the tooth pulp are more densely innervated than less sensitive tissues like muscles or visceral organs.

The pain receptors may be activated by any kind of stimulation. They are, however, normally relatively insensitive to stimulation compared to other types of specific nerve endings in the skin, such as receptors for touch, vibration, pressure or temperature. A relatively strong stimulus is therefore required to activate the pain endings though under certain pathological conditions their sensitivity may increase considerably. This may, for instance, occur during inflammation of a tissue. For example, after sunburn the pain endings in the skin may become extremely sensitive and the slightest touch is then painful. This increase in sensitivity is attributed to the release of pain-inducing substances such as bradykinin, serotonin or prostaglandins into inflamed tissue.

Pain Nerves

Not all nerve fibres conduct signals with the same velocity. The pain endings are the terminals of two distinct groups of sensory fibres, rapidly conducting A-δ fibres and slowly conducting C fibres (see Fig. 1.2). The difference in conduction

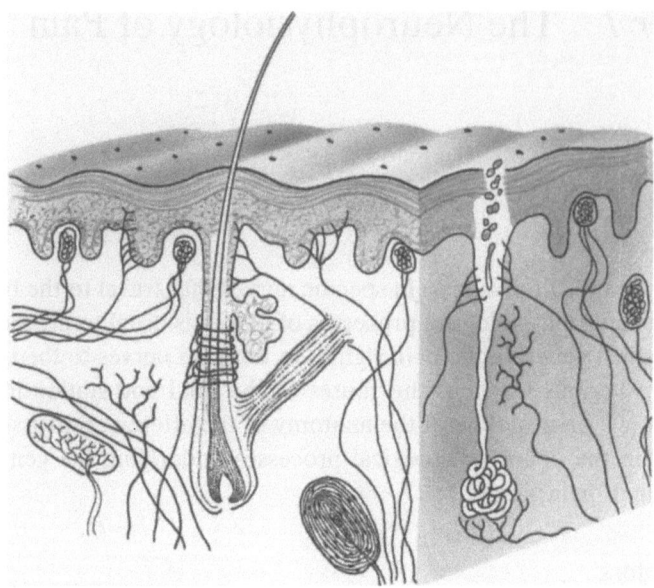

Fig. 1.1. Sensory endings in the skin

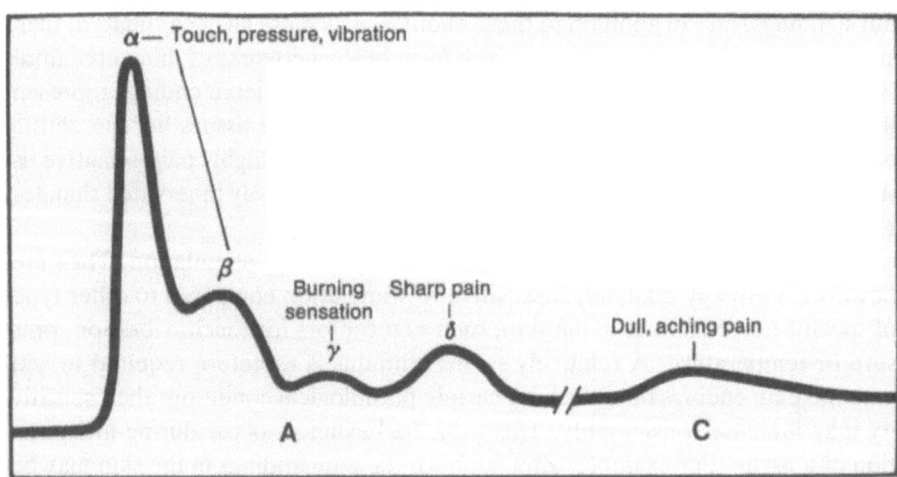

Fig. 1.2. Verbal reports of sensations evoked by stimulation of different groups of afferent fibres

velocity of these two groups explains the phenomenon of double pain. For instance a brief and sharp stimulus to a toe is perceived as coming in two waves, first a sharp sensation of pain which is mediated by the rapidly conducting A-δ fibres and a second wave of dull pain mediated by the slowly conducting C fibres. The pain provoked by stimulation of the A-δ fibres is distinct, sharp, well localized and usually short-lasting while the pain carried by the C fibres is dull, aching, diffuse and generally long-lasting. In clinical practice it is usually the C fibre pain that brings the patient to seek aid. The pain fibres from skin, mucous membranes, muscles and ligaments join the other sensory nerve fibres in their course towards the spinal cord and the brain, whereas the pain fibres from visceral organs pass together with sympathetic and parasympathetic fibres. All pain fibres, like the afferent fibres carrying other sensory signals from the trunk and the extremities, enter the spinal cord through the dorsal roots while the pain fibres from the head pass to the brain stem via the trigeminal nerve.

## Dermatomes and Myotomes

Testing for impairment or loss of cutaneous sensation is an important part of the neurological examination of a patient suffering from pain; it is particulary useful in detecting the site of a lesion involving the spinal cord or nerve roots. The distribution of cutaneous areas (dermatomes) supplied by the spinal nerve is shown in Fig. 1.3a. A dermatomal map that receives general acceptance in all details has yet to be devised since different methods of investigation give different results. Cutaneous areas supplied by adjacent spinal nerves overlap. For example, the upper half of the area supplied by T5 is also supplied by T4, and the lower half by T6. There is therefore little sensory loss, if any, following interruption of a single dorsal root of spinal nerves.

   Reflex contraction of muscles is also used in testing the integrity of segments of the cord and the spinal nerves. The distribution of muscles (myotomes) supplied by the spinal nerve is shown in Fig. 1.3b. The segments involved in the more commonly tested stretch or tendon reflexes are as follows: C5 and C6, biceps reflex; C6, C7 and C8, triceps reflex; L2, L3 and L4, quadriceps reflex; S1 and S2, gastrocnemius reflex.

## Transmission in the Spinal Cord

After entering the spinal cord the pain fibres pass into the dorsal horns where their endings make synaptic contact with second order neurons to which the signals are transmitted (see Fig. 1.4). Until recently the dorsal horns were considered merely as relay stations where the afferent impulses were distributed to different neurons, the axons of which formed ascending pathways to the brain, or mediated spinal reflexes. Recent findings have shown, however, that the neurons of the dorsal horns play a much more important role. Some of these cells may actually act as control neurons which prevent the pain impulses being transmitted to the brain. These control cells may be activated from higher centres in the brain stem, or from subcortical centres, as well as by impulses in large diameter afferent fibres from skin and muscles. The discovery of this control action of the dorsal horn cells forms the basis for the gate control theory which will be discussed later. The pain-relieving effect of TENS is obtained by activation of this physiological control system.

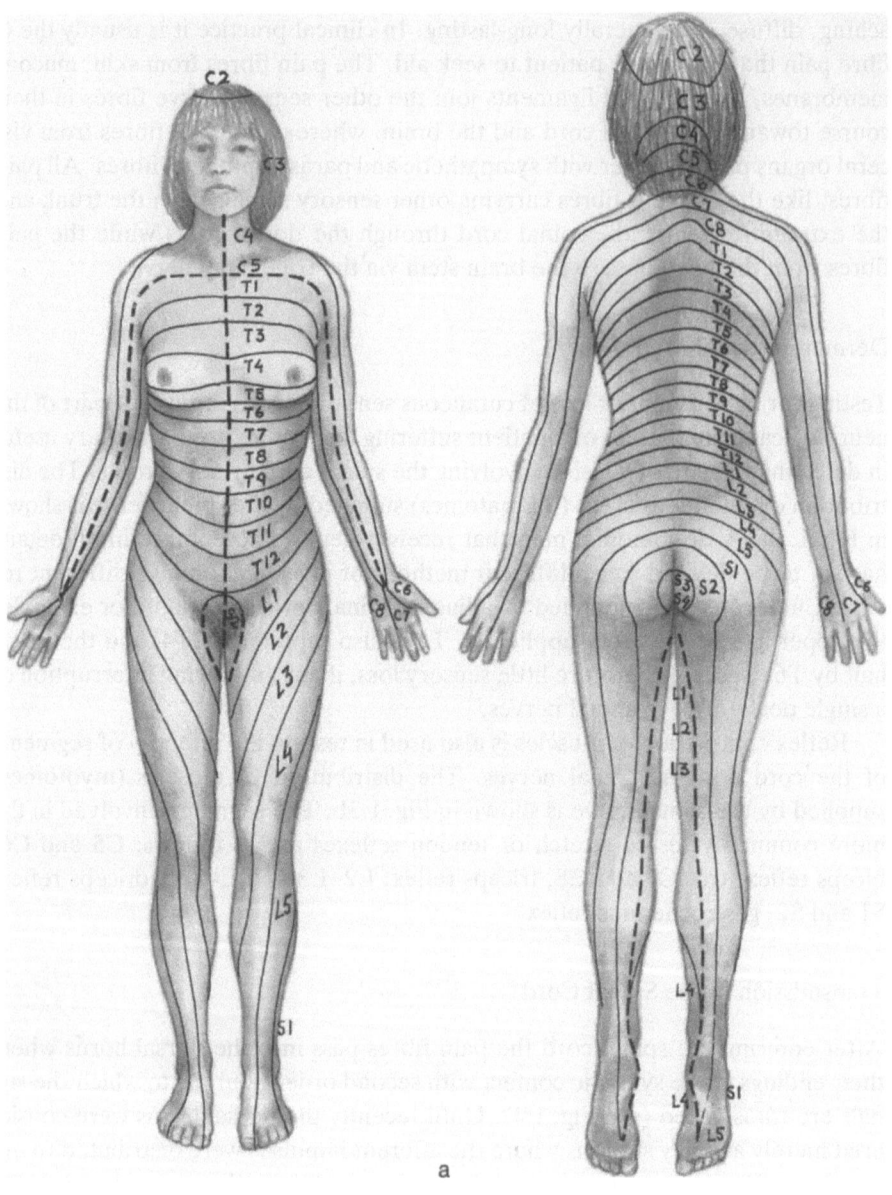

Fig. 1.3. a Dermatomes of the spinal nerves. b, c Myotomes of the skeletal musculature

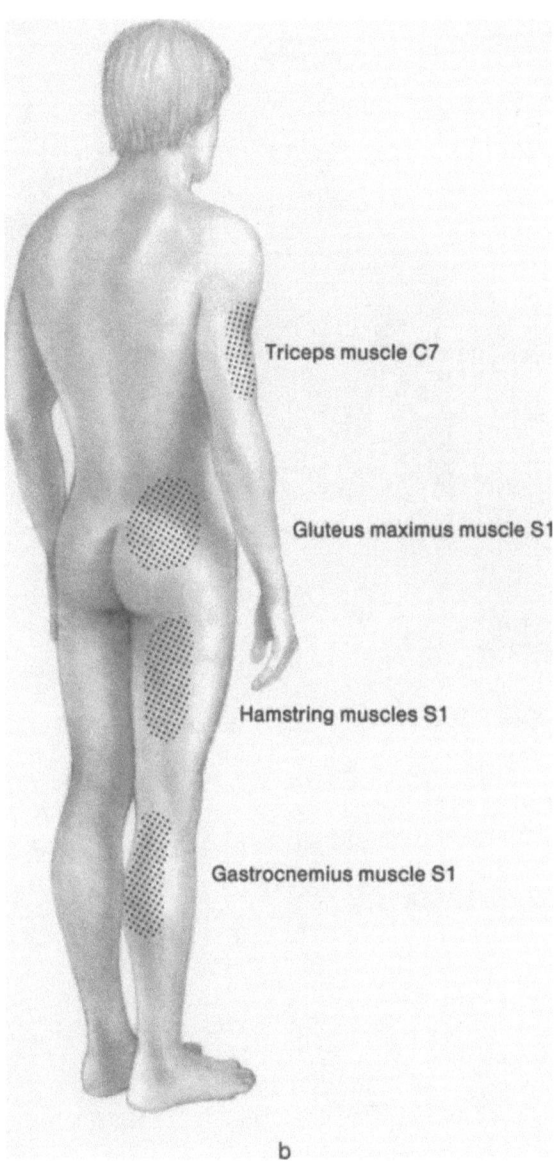

Triceps muscle C7

Gluteus maximus muscle S1

Hamstring muscles S1

Gastrocnemius muscle S1

b

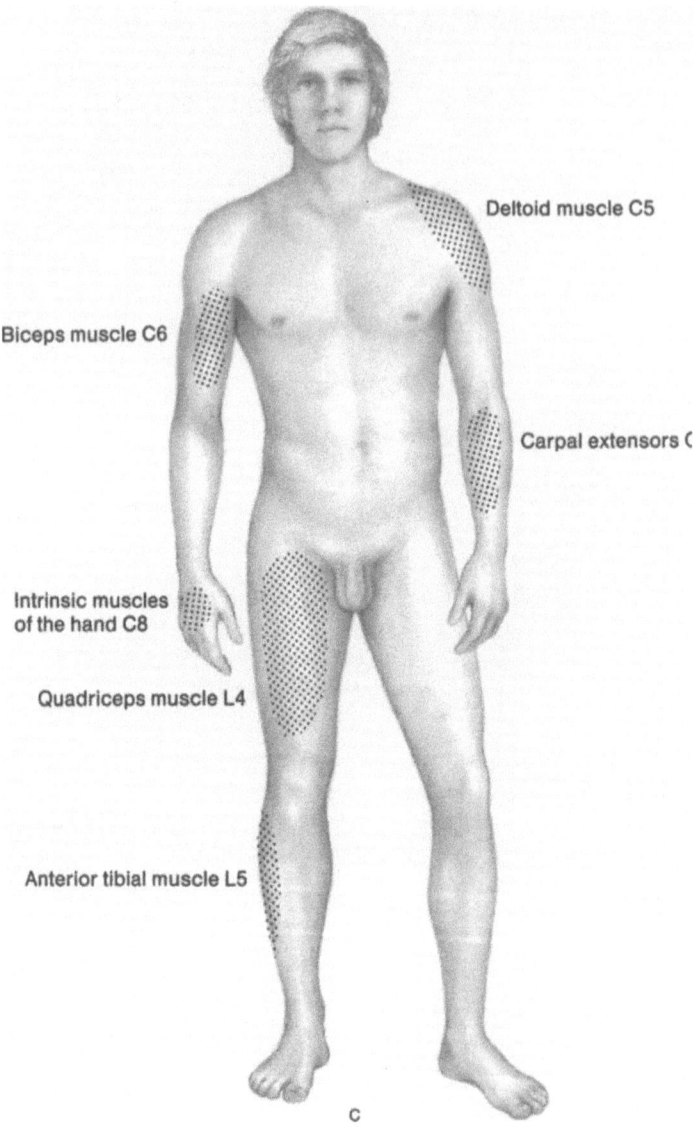

Deltoid muscle C5

Biceps muscle C6

Carpal extensors C

Intrinsic muscles
of the hand C8

Quadriceps muscle L4

Anterior tibial muscle L5

c

Fig. 1.3

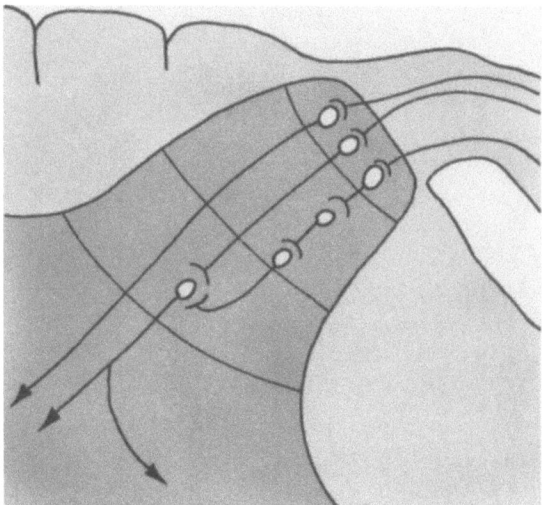

Fig. 1.4. Schematic organization of the dorsal horn of the spinal cord

Ascending Pathways

Pain signals are transmitted to the brain by the axons of certain dorsal horn cells. Most of these axons pass over to the opposite side of the spinal cord and form a pathway, the spinothalamic tract, which ascends in the anterolateral part of the spinal cord (Fig. 1.5). In addition to the spinothalamic tract which forms the principal ascending pain pathway there are several other less well-defined tracts by which pain signals may reach the brain.

When passing through the medulla, the pain fibres of the spinothalamic tract give off numerous collaterals to the respiratory and cardiac centres: painful stimuli through these connections may evoke respiratory and circulatory reflexes. Further on their way to the thalamus they also send branches to centres in the brain stem. Pain signals may have a generally activating action on cortical cells through these latter connections. Before reaching the thalamus the spinothalamic tract divides into two tracts, tractus neospinothalamicus and tractus paleospinothalamicus, which have different end stations in the thalamus. Neurons from the thalamus transmit impulses of the tractus neospinothalamicus to·the somatosensory cortex, while the signals from the paleospinothalamicus are diffusely spread to wider areas of the cortex. The paleospinothalamicus also gives off fibres which spread diffusely deep into the brain before entering the thalamus. It is this projection system that is mainly responsible for the emotional reactions, the anger, fear and suffering which is often associated with the sensation of pain.

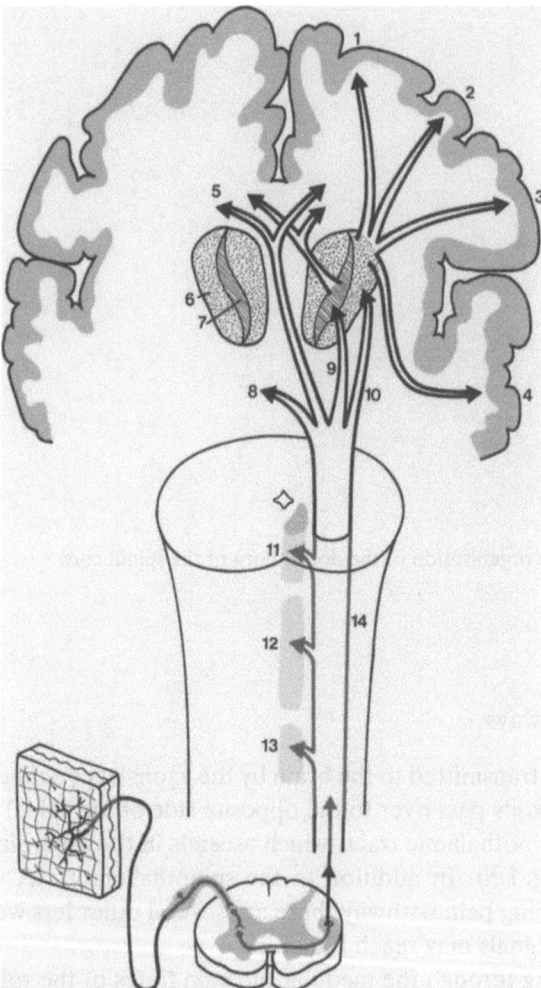

Fig. 1.5. Central projections of the anterolateral spinothalamic pain tract: *1* and *2*, primary somaesthetic areas; *3*, secondary somaesthetic area; *4*, parietal cortex; *5*, projections to the limbic system; *6*, ventrobasal thalamic nuclei; *7*, intrathalamic nuclei; *8*, projection to the hypothalamus; *9*, palaeospinothalamic tract; *10*, neospinothalamic tract; *11*, periaqueductal grey; *12*, reticular formation (medullary part); *13*, cardiac and respiratory medullary centres; *14*, anterolateral spinothalamic tract

## Pain from Different Organ Systems

On the basis of differences in the distribution and density of pain fibres, and in the quality of sensation produced from different tissues, pain can be divided into three categories: pain from skin and superficial tissues, deep somatic pain and visceral pain.

## Pain from the Skin and Superficial Tissues

The quality of pain perception evoked from skin and superficial tissues varies greatly. It may be sharp, pricking, stabbing or burning, short-lived or enduring. In contrast to deep somatic pain and visceral pain, it is, in general, well localised.

Injuries, such as abrasions, burns, freezing, sunburn, etc., may cause an increased sensitivity of the pain endings of the skin. This state is generally referred to as hyperalgesia. The most characteristic feature of this state is the burning quality of the pain. If the injury involves a great area of the skin, the increased sensitivity may extend into surrounding areas which have not been exposed to the injury. This secondary hyperalgesia is supposed to arise from diffusion of substances which are released from the damaged cells in the injured area.

## Deep Somatic Pain

Deep somatic tissues vary greatly in their relative sensitivity to pain-provoking stimuli. Muscle tissue is relatively insensitive while the periostium, ligaments and tendons are highly sensitive to noxious (painful) stimuli. The pain from deep somatic tissues is generally diffuse and is often perceived as coming from a region of the body other than the actual site of provocation.

*Musculoskeletal pain* is the most common form of deep somatic pain. It may arise in several ways, the most common being: (a) prolonged load; (b) impaired blood supply; (c) inflammatory processes; (d) trauma or sudden overload of a muscle or groups of muscles.

The mechanism by which muscle pain arises is poorly understood. Since muscle tissue in general has a very sparse innervation of pain fibres, it is likely that the pain comes mainly from pain endings in muscle tendons, ligaments and fasciae. In inflammatory states the sensitivity of the pain endings is increased by release of pain-producing substances. This is also the likely cause of the pain due to an impaired blood supply. Ischaemic pain has been attributed to the accumulation of metabolic products or other substances such as bradykinin. With prolonged overload the reduced circulation may contribute to pain through similar mechanisms. In pain arising from a sudden overload it appears that mechanical factors such as rupture of ligaments, etc. may be the main factors.

## Visceral Pain

Visceral organs are relatively insensitive to many of the stimuli that provoke intense pain in skin and deep somatic tissues. This is most likely due to the sparse pain innervation of visceral organs. Pain impulses from viscera reach the brain by various routes. Pain fibres from abdominal organs travel to the spinal cord in company with autonomic nerve fibres, whereas those from the inner walls of the abdominal and thoracic cavities accompany somatic nerves. The quality and per-

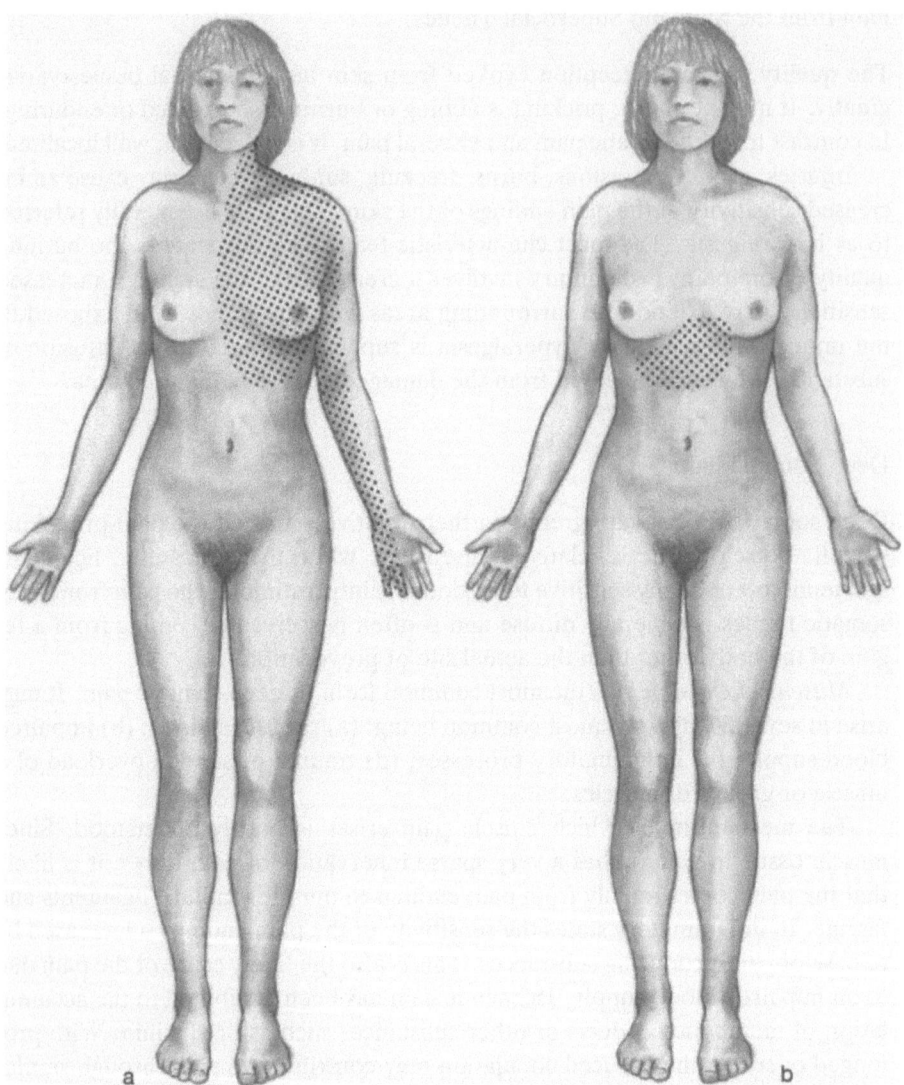

Fig. 1.6a–d. Distribution of referred pain from the heart (a), the *upper part* of the gastrointestinal tract (b), the right urinary tract (c), and the diaphragm (d)

ceived location of the pain arising from visceral organs therefore varies depending on the set of fibres activated.

   In general, pain from visceral organs is diffuse and difficult to localise. Often it is felt as coming from regions other than the actual source. Such pain is said to be "referred" (see below). This is often seen in angina pectoris where, typically, pain radiates to the left shoulder and thence down the left arm to the elbow or the wrist (Fig. 1.6a). Pain arising from the intestinal tract is usually felt diffusely in the midline of the abdomen (see Fig. 1.6b), but pain from the appendix is felt

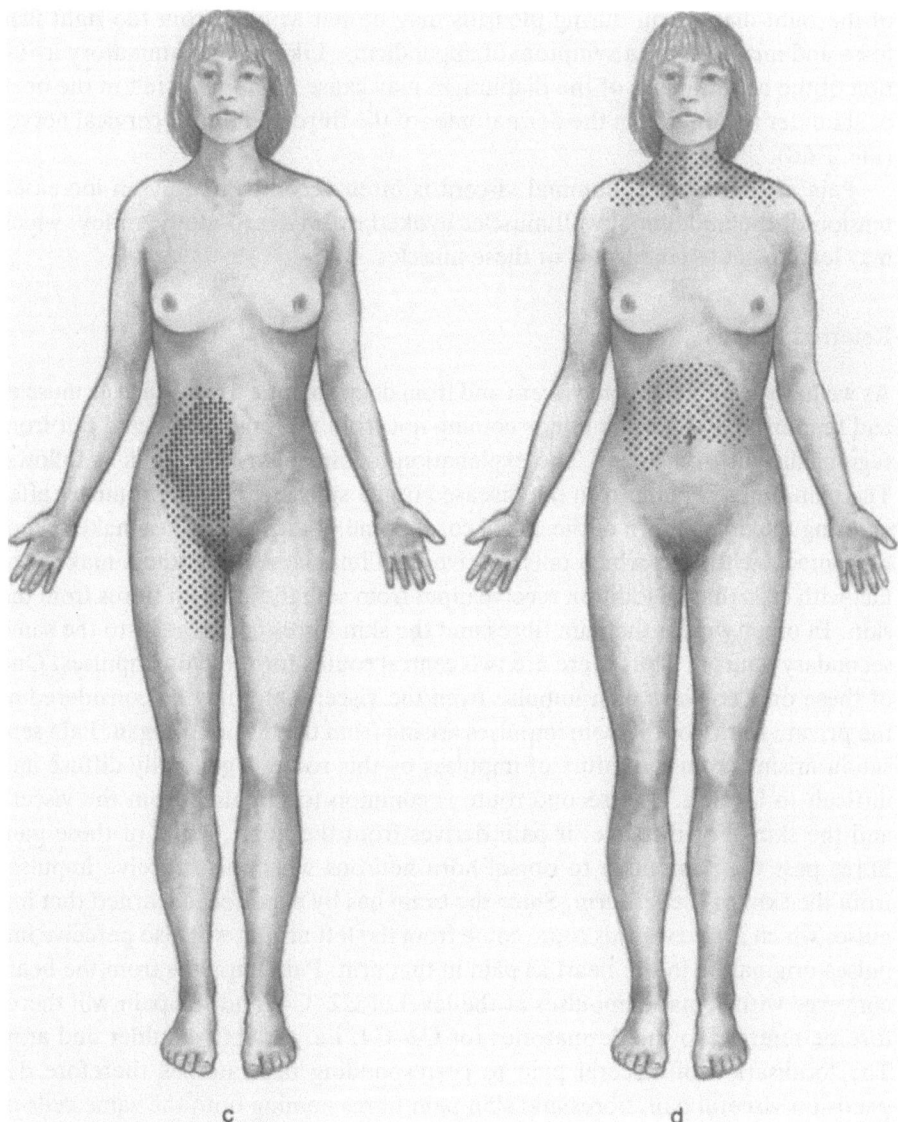

c                                    d

below and to the right of the umbilicus. Pathological processes in the urinary bladder give rise to pain in the suprapubic region whereas pain coming from the ureter or the kidney is referred to the lower half of the abdomen and flank and often radiates to the groin on the affected side (Fig. 1.6c).

When an inflammatory process in a visceral organ spreads to affect the abdominal or thoracic walls so that the pain fibres of these structures are also affected, the pain often becomes more distinct and well localised. However, referred pain may give rise to diagnostic errors. For instance, irritation of the margins of the right diaphragm during pleuritis may be felt as pain from the right iliac fossa and mistaken for a symptom of appendicitis. Likewise inflammatory irritation of the central parts of the diaphragm may cause pain that is felt in the neck or shoulder region within the dermatomes of the third and fourth cervical nerves (Fig. 1.6d).

Pain arising from abdominal viscera is often accompanied by an increased tension of the abdominal wall muscles evoked by a viscero-motor reflex, which may lead to acute tenderness of these muscles.

Referred Pain

As we have seen, pain from viscera and from deep somatic tissues such as muscles and tendons may often be felt as coming not from the organs affected but from regions distant from them. The explanation for this phenomenon is as follows. The pain fibres coming from the diseased organ split into several branches after entering the dorsal horn of the spinal cord. Some of these branches make synaptic contacts with cells which only receive pain impulses while others make contact with cells that in addition receive input from somatic afferent fibres from the skin. In other words, the pain fibres and the skin fibres converge onto the same secondary neuron. Thus there are two central routes for the pain impulses. One of these only conveys pain impulse from the viscera and may be considered as the private route for the pain impulses arising from the diseased organ. Pain sensation arising from the influx of impulses by this route is generally diffuse and difficult to localise. The second route is common to impulses from the viscera and the skin. For instance, if pain derives from the heart, some of these pain fibres pass their impulses to dorsal horn neurons which also receive impulses from the skin of the left arm. Since the brain has by experience learned that impulses which arrive via this route come from the left arm, it will also perceive impulses originating in the heart as pain in that arm. Pain impulses from the heart converge with somatic impulses at the level of C2–C4, and the pain will therefore be referred to the dermatories for C2–C4, i.e. the left shoulder and arm. The localisation of visceral pain to corresponding dermatomes therefore depends on visceral pain fibres and skin pain fibres coming onto the same cells of the dorsal horn.

## Physiological Mechanisms of Pain Control

It is a well-known fact that pain may be blocked by strong emotional reactions. For instance, during the excitment of the game a rugby player may not notice that he has been severely injured. This and similar experiences clearly show that physiological mechanisms exist by which pain may be controlled. Until recently

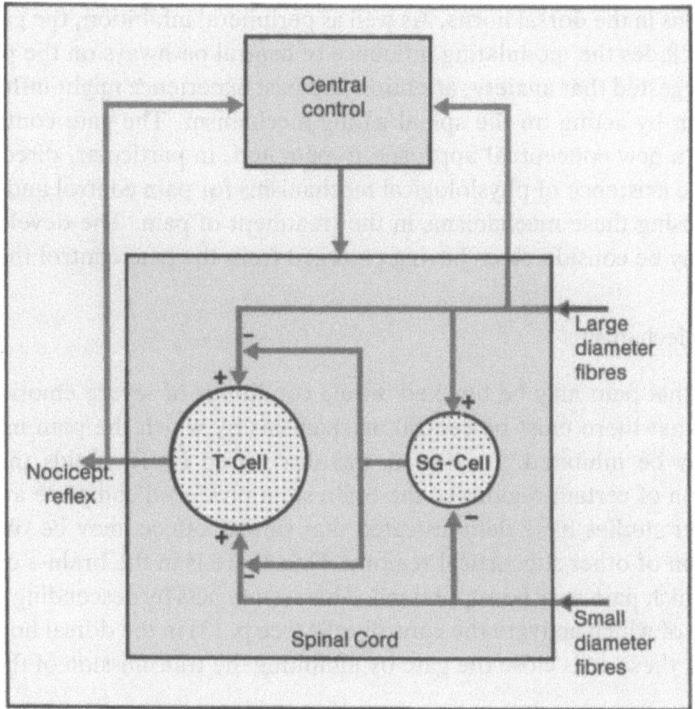

Fig. 1.7. Gate control theory of pain

the neurophysiological processes underlying this control were almost completely unknown. In the last two decades discoveries have been made which have shed light on these control mechanisms. This new knowledge has provided the basis for development of new and powerful methods in combatting pain. In principle these methods, either through a peripheral input or by activating central mechanisms in the brain or brain stem, interrupt or control the transmission of pain impulses.

Peripheral Mechanisms

It is a well-known phenomenon that pain-relieving effects can be obtained from cutaneous stimulation such as massage, vibration or cold applications. Neurophysiological studies show that this may be explained by an interaction between large diameter fibres and pain fibres at the level of the dorsal horns. On the basis of these findings, Melzack and Wall (1965) formulated their well-known theory of a gate control system which controls the input of pain impulses to the brain (Fig. 1.7). According to this theory, activity in afferent large diameter fibres from skin and muscles inhibits the synaptic transmission of pain fibres to secondary neurons in the dorsal horns. As well as peripheral inhibition, the gate control theory includes the modulating influence of central pathways on the pain input. It was suggested that anxiety, attention and past experience might influence pain perception by acting on the spinal gating mechanism. The gate control theory provided a new conceptual approach to pain and, in particular, directed attention to the existence of physiological mechanisms for pain control and the possibility of using these mechanisms in the treatment of pain. The development of TENS may be considered as having emerged from the gate control theory.

Central Mechanisms

The fact that pain may be blocked during conditions of severe emotional stress suggests that there must be central mechanisms by which the pain input to the brain may be inhibited. In 1969 it was discovered by Reynolds that electric stimulation of certain regions of the brain stem produced complete analgesia in rats. Later studies have demonstrated that similar effects may be obtained by stimulation of other subcortical regions. Thus there is in the brain a central system by which pain may be suppressed. This system acts by descending pathways, the fibres of which activate the control cells (see p. 13) in the dorsal horns. When activated, these cells close the gate by inhibiting the transmission of the pain impulses.

An important question is under what conditions this control system exerts its actions. It appears to be activated by afferent input in large diameter fibres from the skin and from muscles or from higher centres. Impulses in these fibres thus (a) directly activate the control cells of the dorsal horns; (b) activate through ascending pathways the pain control centres in the brain stem, which in turn through descending pathways act upon the control cells in the dorsal horns. The brain stem control centres may also be triggered into action through psychological reactions such as anxiety, anger and psychic shock and may then cause a complete elimination of pain. Certain people like yogis appear to be able to turn on this system at will.

Neurohumoral Mechanisms

In 1973 it was discovered by Terenius that opiates and opiate-like drugs exert their pain-relieving effect by binding to specific opiate receptors in the brain. The search for the natural ligands of these receptors led soon thereafter to the demonstration of a family of hitherto unknown peptides which exert an inhibitory action on the transmission of pain impulses in the spinal cord and in the brain. The peptide discovered first was termed enkephalin. Later a number of other peptides with similar properties were identified. These substances were called endorphins. Since none of these substances is able to pass through the blood-brain barrier, they cannot be administered orally or intravenously. Some of them, when administered into the cisterns of the brain, have an analgesic effect which is considerably stronger than that of morphine.

Enkephalin has been found in the neurons of the pain control system. It is generally assumed to be a neurotransmitter which exerts its pain-controlling function by activating control cells of the dorsal horns. Morphine has a molecular configuration which is closely similar to one part of the endorphin molecule. Morphine is therefore assumed to exert its pain-relieving action by binding to the endorphin receptors and thereby activating the pain control system. Additionally morphine has a euphoric effect.

The action of morphine can be counteracted by administering a morphine antagonist, naloxone, which blocks the endorphin receptors, thereby antagonising the endorphin effect. Naloxone by itself has little or no effect in low doses and has therefore been widely used to determine whether or not the pain-relieving effect of a given treatment is mediated by release of endorphin. For instance, the analgesic effect of electrical stimulation of the brain stem may be blocked by naloxone, as is also the pain relief achieved by acupuncture and low-frequency TENS, indicating that these treatments act by releasing endorphin. Pain relief by high-frequency TENS or hypnosis, on the other hand, is not affected by administration of naloxone, which suggests that their analgesic effect is not endorphin mediated.

## References

Melzack R, Wall PD (1965) Pain mechanism: a new theory. Science 150:971
Reynolds DV (1969) Surgery in the rat during electrical analgesia induced by focal brain stimulation. Science 164:444
Terenius L (1973) Characteristics of the "receptor" for narcotic analgesics in synaptic plasma membrane fraction from rat brain. Acta Pharmacol Toxicol 33:377

## Suggested Reading

Besson J-M, Chaduch A (1987) Peripheral and spinal mechanisms of nociception. Physiol Rev 67:67
Cervero F (1985) Visceral nociception: peripheral and central aspects of visceral nociceptive systems. Philos Trans R Soc Lond [Biol] 308:325
Devor M (1984) The pathophysiology and anatomy of damaged nerve. In: Wall PD, Melzack R (eds) Textbook of pain. Churchill Livingstone, Edinburgh, p 49
Dickenson AH, Le Bars D (1987) Supraspinal morphine and descending inhibitions acting on the dorsal horn of the rat. J Physiol 384:81
Fields HL, Basbaum AI (1984) Endogenous pain control mechanisms. In: Wall PD, Melzack R (eds) Textbook of pain. Churchill Livingstone, Edinburgh, p 142
North AR (1986) Opioid receptor types and membrane ion channels. Trends Neurosci March: 114
Lynn B (1984) The detection of injury and tissue damage. In: Wall PD, Melzack R (eds) Textbook of pain. Churchill Livingstone, Edinburgh, p 19
Terenius L (1984) The endogenous opioids and other central peptides. In: Wall PD, Melzack R (eds) Textbook of pain. Churchill Livingstone, Edinburgh, p 133
Torebjörk HE, Schady W, Ochoa J (1984) Sensory correlates of somatic afferent fibre activation. Hum Neurobiol 3:15

Vallbo ÅB, Hagbarth K-E, Torebjörk HE, Wallin BG (1979) Somatosensory proprioceptive
   and sympathetic activity in human peripheral nerves. Physiol Rev 59:919
Wiesenfeld-Hallin Z, Hallin RG (1984) The influence of the sympathetic system on
   mechanoreception and nociception. Hum Neurobiol 3:41
Willis WD (1982) Control of nociceptive transmission in the spinal cord. In: Ottoson D (ed)
   Sensory physiology 3. Springer, Berlin Heidelberg New York, p 1
Willis WD (1985) The pain system: the neural basis of nociceptive transmission in the mamma-
   lian nervous system (Pain and headache, vol 8). Karger, Basel, p 78

# *Chapter 2* Transcutaneous Electrical Nerve Stimulation

## Introduction

The first modern stimulator for TENS of peripheral nerves for the management of pain was originally developed as a screening device to determine the potential usefulness of surgical implantation of electrodes for the stimulation of the dorsal column of the spinal cord. In these screening tests it became apparent that peripheral stimulation in itself provided excellent pain relief in some patients, and very soon this technique came into widespread use.

At the present time a great number of such stimulators are available with differing electrical characteristics. Evaluation of their properties and usefulness in pain relief is generally based on empirical tests, and there is still a lack of precise knowledge of which stimulus parameters are the most suitable in different pain syndromes. For this reason it is possible to provide only general guidelines of stimulus parameters in using the wide variety of stimulators at present available on the market.

## General Principles for the Use of TENS

A thorough physical examination of the patient in order to arrive at an accurate diagnosis is essential before application of TENS. It is also important to keep in mind the fact that TENS does not cure the disease or dysfunction underlying the pain. Before applying TENS, an evaluation should be made of the characteristics of the pain, its quality, location and temporal features, previous treatment and medication, drug dependency, etc. When applying TENS it should be noted that the source of the pain may sometimes be distant from the site where the patient claims it hurts. A typical example of this is angina pectoris which may be experienced as pain in the left arm. Such referred pain is also common in myofascial pain syndromes. An accurate diagnosis is thus essential for the placement of the electrodes at the optimal sites. For the selection of these sites it is therefore necessary to know the anatomical distribution of dermatomes and myotomes (see pp. 4–6).

For the evaluation of the pain symptom complex, it is often advantageous to use numerical or verbal scales and pain descriptor word lists (see below). The patient should be asked to outline the spatial distribution of pain and indicate the region of most intense pain. Such a chart may be useful in evaluating the effect following TENS. Assessment should also be made of sensory loss, range of movement, gait and posture for later evaluation of the effect of TENS.

Of the different modes of stimulation offered by commercial TENS units, conventional high-frequency (50–100 Hz) stimulation is always the first mode to be tried. The potential benefit of this mode of stimulation is critically dependent on the correct placement of the electrodes. If no pain relief is obtained after 20–30 min of stimulation, different placements of the electrodes should be tried. If stimulation is unsuccessful after the evaluation of various electrode arrangements, either low-frequency pulse-train or intense low-frequency acupuncture-like stimulation should be tried. Note that in changing to these modes of stimulation a different electrode placement may be required. Furthermore, stimulus intensity should be increased until strong rhythmic muscle contractions are elicited.

The induction time for maximal pain relief with either of these two modes of stimulation is generally 20–30 min or longer. Stimulation should therefore be continued for at least 30 min before the effect can be assessed.

Quantitative assessment of the outcome of TENS treatment encounters the difficulty that pain is a subjective experience and as such difficult to measure. However, different pain measurement scales exist which may be used in order to obtain an objective evaluation of the treatment outcome. The simplest of these scales uses a four or five point descriptive scale based on the patient's experience of the pain intensity: (a) no pain; (b) moderate; (c) severe; (d) very severe; (e) unbearable. Another is the numerical rating scale. This scale uses numbers from 0 to 10, and the patient is asked to indicate the intensity of his pain in terms of a number, 0 indicating no pain and 10 unbearable pain. A third scale, the visual analogue scale, is similar to the numerical scale, but without the division into ten units. It consists of a 10-cm line, and the patient is asked to place a mark at a point along the line that represents the intensity of his pain, the ends of the line indicating no pain and unbearable pain, respectively. Whatever scale is used to evaluate the effect of TENS treatment the intensity of the pain should be assessed immediately before and after the treatment.

In all evaluations of the pain relief of TENS the placebo response should be taken into account. The placebo response is the reaction of a patient that has no causative relation to the type of intervention used and may be attributed to the patient's hope or expectations of treatment success. It has been estimated (Thorsteinsson et al. 1978) that about 30% of the initial successful outcomes of TENS trials can be accounted for by placebo responses. In general, placebo responses diminish rapidly with repeated treatments and may disappear completely in most patients after 1 month. A safe assessment of the TENS effect can therefore not be made before a number of treatments have been carried out over a period of at least 1 month.

It is a general observation that the pain-relieving effect of TENS in treating chronic pain falls off with time. A proportion of the early reduction in pain relief may therefore be accounted for by the placebo phenomenon. However, also for patients who continue to use TENS for months, there is a gradual decrease in the efficacy of TENS. In the long term it has been found (Eriksson et al. 1979) that only 20%–30% of chronic pain patients still continue to use the device after 1 year, for instance. The cause of the decline in efficacy of TENS treatment is not known. To reduce and delay this decrease, alternating electrode placement may be tried. Again, if TENS treatment is discontinued for a period of time (during which some other physical treatment may be tried) and then resumed, there is evidence that the pain-relieving effect can be enhanced.

## Indications for the Use of TENS

TENS as treatment of pain is unique in the sense that it exerts its pain-relieving effect by activating built-in control mechanisms of the nervous system. It is consequently non-hazardous, non-invasive, non-addictive and practically without side effects. It is therefore not surprising that TENS has become a widely used method for treatment of pain. The enthusiasm following the first reports of TENS, which claimed success in 80%–100% of a variety of pain syndromes, resulted in its indiscriminate use. Following more prolonged studies and placebo controls it became obvious that TENS treatment was not a panacea, and that its pain-relieving effect often declined rapidly with time.

Although TENS is effective in treating acute pain, its major role is in the management of chronic pain. TENS is particularly beneficial in the treatment of chronic low back pain, myofascial pain syndromes, pain of neurogenic origin and peripheral nerve injury, pain secondary to rheumatoid arthritis and the pain of spinal injury. TENS has also been used with varying degrees of success in the treatment of post-herpetic neuralgia, phantom limb pain, headache, and cancer pain. In some chronic pain states such as psychogenic pain and central pain TENS is likely to offer little pain relief except for the placebo response.

Recent studies show that TENS is effective for treatment of acute pain and particularly for managing pain following surgery (see post-operative pain, pp. 41–44). TENS has also been used with success in relieving acute pain due to non-musculoskeletal trauma such as muscle spasms and ligamentous strains in athletes. In these cases TENS should be used with caution and not in order to allow the athlete to go back to play, thereby exposing himself to the risk of aggravating the injury.

## General Characteristics of TENS Units

Although the commercially available transcutaneous electrical stimulators may differ in their stimulating characteristics, they have some features in common. Most devices allow the clinician or the patient to vary the stimulus intensity, pulse rate and pulse width. In some models the pulse width may be fixed and only the stimulus intensity variable. At present most commercial TENS units are designed to deliver short pulses at a regular rate which is adjustable (Fig. 2.1). However, the configuration of these pulses may vary greatly from one device to another. Most units have a single-channel output although some may have dual-channel output. Many TENS units deliver a constant current output at a given setting of stimulus intensity. In evaluating the efficiency of different models of TENS units, it is particularly important to take this feature into account.

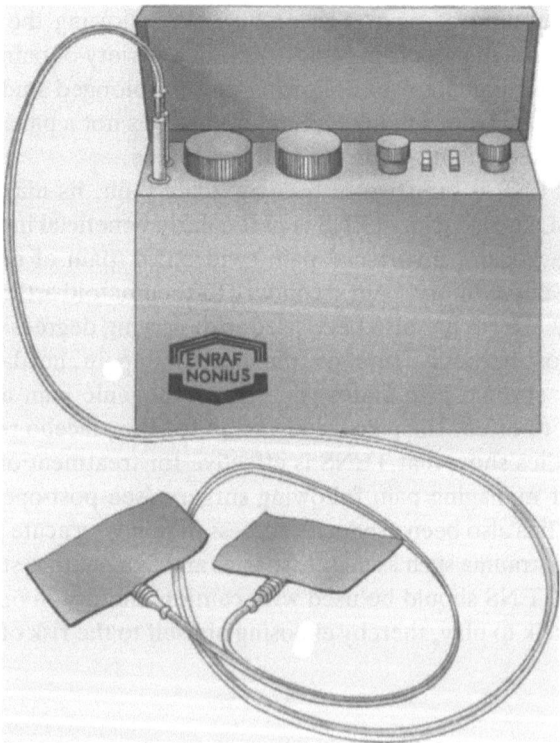

Fig. 2.1. TENS unit with electrodes

# Conventional High-Frequency TENS

## Stimulus Intensity

In all stimulators, irrespective of the waveform they deliver, the amplitude of the electrical pulses can be varied. Large diameter nerve fibres have lower thresholds for excitation than small nerve fibres, and a gradual increase of the stimulus amplitude from zero will therefore first excite fibres of large diameter and, with increasing strength, smaller and smaller fibres. Since the basic principle of TENS for pain relief is to excite more or less exclusively the spectrum of large diameter fibres, the correct amplitude setting of the stimulator is essential. Empirically it has been found that the amplitude of the stimulating pulses should be increased to a level at which the stimulus is experienced as just beginning to be uncomfortable, but below the pain threshold. When properly adjusted the stimulation should create a sensation of tingling or pricking which should not be unpleasant. It is assumed that at this strength the stimulus is activating the entire spectrum of large diameter fibres and some medium-sized fibres (Wall and Sweet 1967).

During a stimulation session, which lasts between 30 min to several hour, the tingling or pricking sensation may gradually fade away. The diminished effect of the stimulus is due to the adaptation of the nerve fibres. To obtain an optimal effect of treatment, it is therefore necessary to adjust the amplitude of the stimulus during the session so as to preserve the tingling, pricking sensation.

The electrical resistance of the skin and underlying tissues to the current delivered by the stimulator is an important factor that may influence the efficiency of the stimulus. This resistance varies with conditions such as skin temperature, peripheral circulation, size of the electrodes and the sort of conductive gel used. To minimise the effect of these variables, most types of commercial stimulators are now designed to deliver a constant current. The voltage output of these stimulators varies automatically to compensate for differences in electrode-skin resistance and thus maintain a constant current output.

## Frequency

Pulse frequency is another important parameter in optimising stimulation. For large diameter sensory fibres the normal range of frequency of firing is 50–100 Hz. At rates higher than 100 Hz they tend to become fatigued after a while. Increasing the frequency above 100 Hz does not therefore enhance the pain-relieving effect of stimulation. The optimal stimulus frequency for activation of large diameter fibres over a period of 30–60 min is therefore in the range 50–100 Hz. It should be noted that small fibres are unable to fire at these rates, and when stimulated at frequencies above 5–10 Hz, most small fibres rapidly become exhausted. The optimal frequency for TENS has not been unequivocally determined, but studies suggest that frequencies from 50 to 100 Hz are the most efficient. This has been termed "high-frequency conventional TENS stimulation" "acupuncture-like" in contrast to "low-frequency stimulation" (see below) (Eriksson and Sjölund 1976; Wall and Sweet 1967).

## Polarity

When an electrical stimulus is applied to the skin, the current passes into the underlying tissue from one electrode to another. For stimulators delivering monophasic rectangular pulses one electrode (usually marked black) represents the negative pole (cathode) while the other (usually marked red) represents the positive pole (anode). Activation of the nerve fibres takes place at the negative pole, and the positive pole (for the current strengths used with TENS) may be regarded as the inactive pole. In placing the electrodes it is therefore important that the negative electrode is placed at an appropriate site, particularly when the stimulus is aimed at peripheral nerve trunks. In searching for the optimal site, several placements of the negative electrode should be tried until the best site is found.

For TENS units delivering symmetric biphasic or asymmetric biphasic pulses, both electrodes are active and will excite underlying nerves. Therefore different placements of both electrodes have to be tried when such units are used.

## Pulse Width

The pulse width is an important parameter of the stimulus since, for a given setting of the amplitude of the stimulating pulses, the spectrum of fibres activated depends on the width of the pulse wave. The general rule is that the shorter the pulse duration, the greater the amplitude required to activate a given set of nerve fibres. For a given width of the stimulating pulses, large diameter fibres are excited at a lower amplitude of the stimulus than small fibres. In order to obtain optimal pain relief, it is essential to activate mainly the large diameter fibres. The correct pulse width setting is crucial when using stimulators which allow variations of pulse width. In many stimulators the pulse width has a fixed duration (usually 0.2 ms) in order to eliminate problems in adjusting the amplitude for varied settings of pulse duration.

## Waveform

Most modern stimulators offer electrical pulses of various waveforms (Fig. 2.2). Some devices may produce symmetrical biphasic rectangular pulses, sine wave pulses, triangular pulses, spike-like pulses, etc. No systematic analysis has been carried out on the relative efficiency of the various waveforms in different pain syndromes, and it is therefore not possible to determine the most effective pulse configuration.

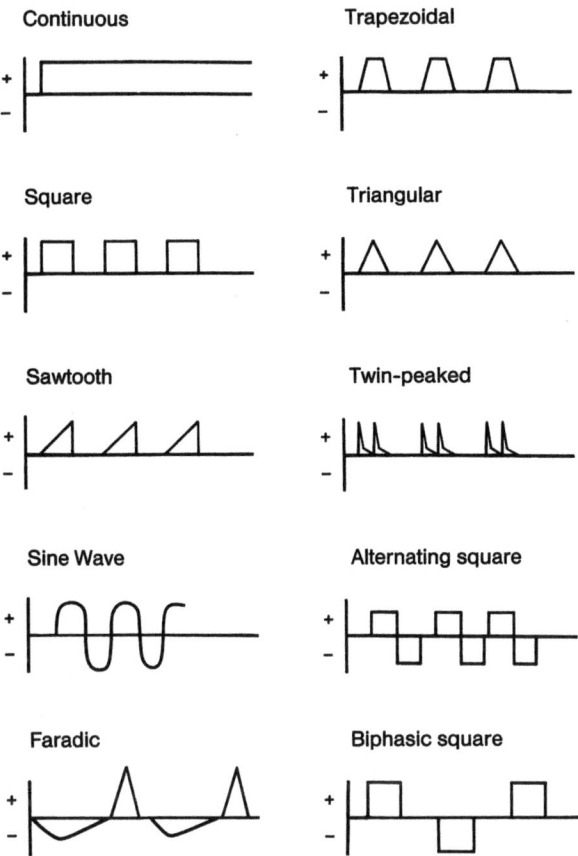

Fig. 2.2. Characteristics of different stimulating waveforms

Battery Charging

Most TENS units are equipped with a 9-V NiCd rechargeable battery. It is charged by connecting the battery charger to a jack on the stimulator without opening the unit. The stimulator should be charged before its first use. With normal usage it is usually sufficient to recharge every 2nd or 3rd day. Recharging takes 10–14 h during which time the stimulator should be switched off. Most stimulators can be used with a 9-V alkaline (transistor) battery. It is important to remember that a TENS unit with such a battery should under no circumstances be recharged.

## Alternative Modes of TENS

### Low-Frequency TENS

In low-frequency TENS, stimulus parameters similar to those in electro-acupuncture are used. This mode of stimulation is also known as "acupuncture-like TENS". To obtain pain relief, high-intensity stimulation is required at a rate of 1–4 Hz and with a pulse width of 0.15–0.25 ms. The stimulation should be intense enough to produce visible muscle contractions in order to be effective. In general the pain-relieving effect does not appear until after 20–30 min of stimulation. Following cessation of stimulation there is a period of post-stimulative pain relief which generally lasts longer than with conventional TENS. A major problem with this kind of TENS is that the muscle contractions may initially increase the pain and so is not well-tolerated by the patients.

### Low-Frequency Pulse-Train TENS

This type of stimulation was developed by applying the principles used in Chinese electro-acupuncture. When first introduced by Eriksson and Sjölund in 1976, it was called "electro-acupuncture", but to avoid confusion with classical electrical acupuncture stimulation, it was later known as "low-frequency pulse-train stimulation" or "pulse-train burst stimulation". This mode delivers impulses at a rate of about 2 Hz (with an inner train frequency of about 80 Hz) instead of pulses at a regular rate (Fig. 2.3). When using this mode of stimulation, it is important to note that the stimulus intensity should be increased until mus-

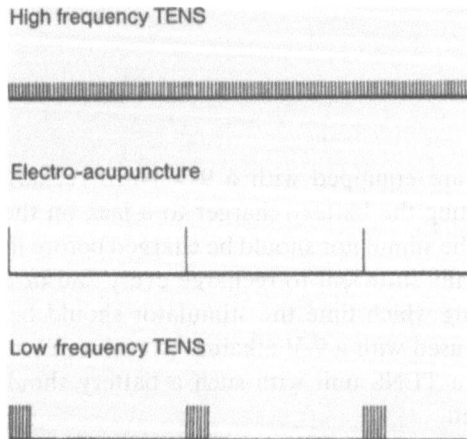

Fig. 2.3. Different methods of TENS. High-frequency stimulation involving continuous barrage of brief pulses. Electro-acupuncture involving single brief pulses. Low-frequency train stimulation consisting of short trains of brief pulses at slow repetition rate. Pulse amplitude indicates differences in stimulus intensity with the three types of stimulation

cle contractions are obtained. In patients who do not respond to conventional high-frequency TENS, this low-frequency type of stimulation has often helped. Several commercial stimulators now offer both stimulus modes.

In using TENS for patients with chronic pain, it is advisable to start with conventional high-frequency TENS. If this does not give satisfactory results (after careful testing of different electrode locations), low-frequency pulse-train TENS could be tried. It should be noted, however, that the most effective electrode placements for low-frequency TENS are sometimes not the same as for high-frequency TENS (see pp. 21–23).

Intense TENS

Various modes of "intense" stimulation have been introduced. In one of these methods, stimulation is applied at a rate of 100–150 Hz, a wide pulse width of 0.5–1 ms and at the highest tolerable intensity. This mode of stimulation produces monorhythmical muscle contractions. Placement of the electrodes close to the painful area is recommended. With this method electro-analgesia may be achieved in 1–15 min, but this effect vanishes when stimulation is ended. In another of these methods stimulation is applied at low frequency (4 Hz) and high intensity (25 times the perception threshold). This mode, as the previous mode, produces local rhythmical muscle contractions. Contrary to most other modes of intense TENS, this mode is without undue discomfort to the patient and may produce long-lasting alleviation of pain (Pomeranz 1987).

# The Neural Mechanisms of TENS in Alleviating Pain

It has been demonstrated in studies on cats and rats (Wall and Melzack 1984) that peripheral activation of large diameter fibres selectively inhibits the transmission of pain impulses in the dorsal horn of the spinal cord and thereby prevents pain input to the brain. In addition to activating local inhibitory circuits in the dorsal horn, stimulation of large diameter fibres seems to activate specific pain control centres in the brain stem which, by descending pathways, controls the pain input to higher centres.

There is a great deal of evidence (Wall and Melzack 1984) that endogenous opioids are involved in pain suppression; for instance, enkephalin-containing neurones are present in the dorsal horn. Although many aspects of pain modulation by endogenous opioids remain unclear, there is nevertheless strong evidence that these opioids play a role in the pain relief obtained with TENS.

## Electrodes and Electrode Placements

### Stimulating Electrodes

When TENS was first introduced, a variety of different types of electrodes was used. At present most stimulators are equipped with carbon rubber electrodes which are reusable and can be fixed to the skin with adhesive tape. Generally they are easily adaptable to the contour of the body region to be stimulated. However, electrodes are sometimes rather stiff and do not always mould well around body contours. They then tend to become loose and air spaces easily develop between electrodes and the skin. Most kinds of electrodes require the application of a conductive gel. One of their disadvantages is that some patients may develop an allergy to the gel, particularly with repeated applications over periods of weeks or months. Before application of the gel the skin area receiving the electrode should be cleaned with mild soap and water and dried thoroughly. If electrodes are kept in place for long periods ($> 4$h) there is a possibility of the conductive gel drying.

Most manufacturers of TENS units supply electrodes of different sizes and shapes to be used with their devices. When selecting suitable electrodes for treatment, it is important to know that the current density is greater with small electrodes than with large ones. If pain is spread over a large area, a pair of small electrodes may not provide efficient stimulation. In such cases multiple pairs of small electrodes or one pair of large electrodes may be used. Note that the efficiency of large electrodes is not directly proportional to their size. Sometimes electrodes of unequal sizes provide the best effect.

In recent years pre-gelled electrodes have become available. These electrodes are generally self-adhering with an adhesive area around the stimulating surface. It has been reported that the incidence of skin irritation with this kind of electrode is less than that observed with carbon rubber electrodes and conventional gels. Many types of self-adhesive electrodes require only water for conduction and are therefore to be recommended to patients for TENS treatment at home. These electrodes are also very useful when testing various placements.

Most types of disposable electrodes are non-sterile, but may be sterilised in an autoclave and stored in airtight envelopes for later use. Sterile pre-gelled and self-adhesive electrodes specially manufactured for treatment of acute postoperative pain are now available. Most of these electrodes have large stimulating surfaces and are rectangular in shape for placement parallel to the incision.

### Electrode Placements

The placement of the electrodes at optimal stimulation sites is perhaps the most important step in applying TENS. There are unfortunately few studies on the effectiveness of different electrode placements in the literature, although some basic principles in the selection of electrode sites have emerged which could serve as guidelines (Gersh and Woolf 1985; Laitinen 1976; Lampe 1978; Linzer and Long 1976; Mannheimer 1978; Woolf 1984; Woolf et al. 1981).

The optimal sites vary from one patient to another even if the symptoms of pain are similar. In each patient it is therefore important to examine carefully the effectiveness of stimulating different sites in order to find out those which are optimal. It is best to begin by placing the electrodes in or around the area of pain, unless there are specific counterindications for this (see below). Even if the first trial gives a positive response, other placements and stimulating parameters should be tried in order to determine the optimal sites and stimulating conditions. This may require treatments over a period of several days. A basic prerequisite for successful TENS treatment is that the patient has adequate cutaneous sensation in the area where the electrodes are placed. If this is not the case, other sites should be tried (see Post-herpetic Neuralgia).

In many pain syndromes the painful area is confined to one or more dermatomes, and the optimal stimulating sites may be located within an appropriate dermatome. In general a dermatome corresponds to the underlying myotome, but there are exceptions which it is important to know, particularly when stimulating with low-frequency acupuncture-like or burst TENS. For instance, in the chest it should be noted that the anterior and posterior parts of a dermatome are innervated by different branches of the same spinal nerve. To obtain the maximum pain reduction, both the anterior and posterior portions of the dermatome should be stimulated. When pain derives from irritation of a spinal root and radiates as in sciatic pain, it is recommended that one electrode is placed paraspinally at the appropriate spinal cord level and the other peripherally over the corresponding dermatome. For instance, in sciatic pain involving L5-S1, one electrode may be placed paravertebrally L5-S1 and other over the popliteal space of the same dermatome.

In many pain syndromes the best effect may be obtained by stimulating peripheral nerves at certain superficial points along their course. It is important to know the points at which the nerves are most readily accessible to surface electrodes. This is, for instance, important in the treatment of facial pain syndromes. The trigeminal nerve has three main branches with specific anatomical distribution, and to obtain the optimum effect it is essential to stimulate the branch innervating the painful area.

In treating the pain of peripheral nerve injury, electrodes should be placed proximal to the lesion; if placed distal to the lesion, stimulation may result in increased pain.

Modern TENS devices offer a dual- or multi-channel system for the use of four or more electrodes. These units permit the simultaneous treatment of many points within a painful area which might be useful, particularly if this area is wide or if pain is radiating. Such units are useful when treating conditions like chronic low back pain.

Arrangement of the electrodes may be unilateral or bilateral. Unilateral placement on the side where pain occurs is the most common. Electrodes are in this case placed on one side of the spine, the face, the head, etc. In some pain syndromes such as post-herpetic neuralgia (see pp. 79–81), stimulation cannot be applied over the painful area since this increases the pain. Unilateral stimulation of the contralateral dermatomes may be beneficial in these cases.

Dual-channel and multi-channel units also provide a variety of possible electrode arrangements which may be useful in treating certain pain states. Electrodes can also be tried in areas distant from the source of pain if trials with conventional placements appear unsuccessful. Usually stronger stimulation is then needed to obtain pain relief.

Specific Stimulation Sites

In selection of optimal sites for electrode placement it is often advantageous to place the electrodes at so-called specific points. There are three types of these points: motor points, trigger points and acupuncture points. It is interesting to note that many of these points are located at identical or nearly similar anatomical sites (Fig. 2.4). It has also been demonstrated that there is often a decreased skin resistance at these points and they are therefore particularly suitable for electrical stimulation.

The small region where nerve fibres and blood vessels enter a muscle is the anatomical motor point. The motor points can be identified as palpably tender points in some muscles. Motor points provide particularly suitable electrode sites for low-frequency TENS aimed at evoking muscle contraction.

Trigger points, in contrast to motor points, are not only found in muscles but also in tendons, ligaments and joint capsules. Both motor points and trigger points can be localised by palpation since they are characterised by tenderness. While a motor point represents a well-defined anatomical entity, there is no agreement as to the development or anatomical specialisation of trigger points. Two types of trigger points have been distinguished by Travell and Rinzler (1952): active and latent. An active trigger point is a tender site in a muscle or other tissue that causes the patient pain at rest, while a latent trigger point causes no pain with daily activities, but is tender when palpated.

Pressure or needling at either trigger or acupuncture points produces a deep aching feeling which in Chinese acupuncture literature is called "de Qi". Recent evidence (Wang et al. 1985) suggests that the de Qi sensation may in part be due to a local muscle reflex that grips the needle when it penetrates the muscle at an acupuncture point. Why this deep aching feeling is felt at some muscle sites and not others is, however, not entirely explained. It is possible that the underlying pathological process is also responsible for the basis of the unpleasant feeling produced by pressure or needling apart from local muscle reflexes. The nature of de Qi is still not fully understood. Some myofascial trigger points, particularly those found in the lower regions of the back, are associated with definite nodules of fibrous tissue. These nodules may develop after virus infections or other fever-producing diseases. It has also been suggested (Travell and Simmons 1983) that trigger points develop during the course of growth as a result of musculo-skeletal stresses and strains, particularly those associated with the muscles of the back. These trigger areas are characterised by abnormal vasomotor and sudomotor activity. It is therefore not surprising that trigger points at the chest and back are rare in infants and common in adults. The widespread distribution of trigger points associated with referred pain patterns suggests that both inflammation processes and muscular strains play a role in this aetiology.

Areas where blood vessels and nerves lie close to the surface, rather than hidden under muscles and other tissues, are particularly prone to the formation of trigger points. While the genesis of trigger points is not explained, it is clear that they are commonly found. It is further evident that many trigger points, those due to musculo-skeletal stresses and strains, are invariably found at specific sites.

Abnormal input from muscles, tendons or joints — due to sprain, strain, excessive stretch, injury, or other unusual activity — may summate with activity from trigger points and produce different patterns of referred pain.

## Side Effects and Counterindications of TENS

The most common side effect with TENS treatment is allergic skin reaction. This occurs in approximately 10% of patients. The strongest reaction is usually around the adhesive which keeps the electrodes in place. The TENS treatment can often be continued after changing the adhesive and instructing the patient to have the electrodes in place only while stimulation is under way. Where patients are allergic to the adhesive tape, the electrodes can be kept in place by elastic bands or elastic bandages. These patients may also find self-adhesive electrodes suitable. Allergic reactions can occur, though more rarely, to the electrode paste or to the actual silicone rubber electrodes. When the allergy is to the paste, one has to proceed by trial and error. Allergies to the rubber electrodes can be dealt with by using foam rubber electrodes, moistened with water.

All forms of powerful electric stimulation of the skin can cause burns. This can be avoided by ensuring that the contact surface between the electrode and the skin is well covered with paste (the better the contact, the lower the resistance). Patients with reduced skin sensitivity run the greatest risk of being burnt. Burns can be avoided among these patients by lowering frequency stimulation to its lowest possible effective level — approximately 50 Hz — or by treating the patient with low-frequency TENS. Low-frequency TENS transmits considerably lower amounts of energy to the skin than high-frequency. Examination before a TENS test, and instructions on skin care and electrode application are simple measures to avoid skin irritation and burns.

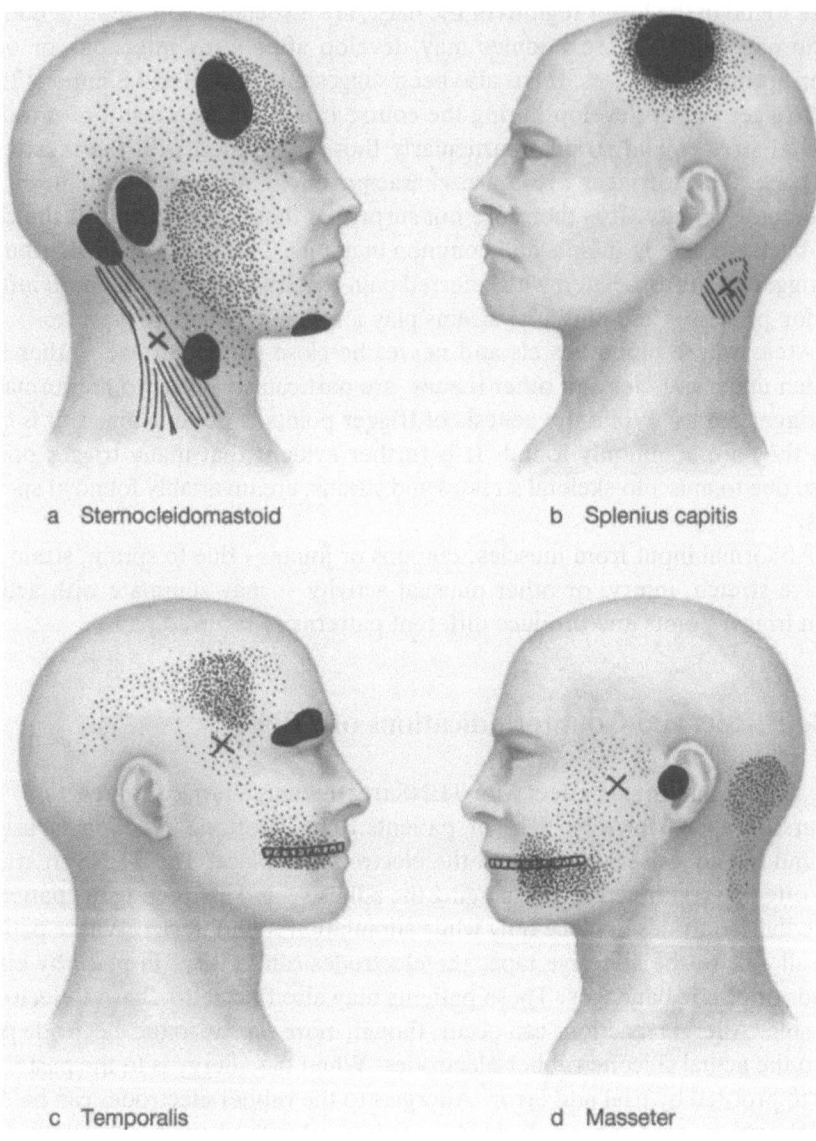

a  Sternocleidomastoid                    b  Splenius capitis

c  Temporalis                             d  Masseter

Fig. 2.4a–w. Location of trigger and acupuncture points *(cross)* associated with myofascial pain syndromes. Pain patterns *(black and strippled areas)*. Muscles affected: (a) Sternocleidomastoid; (b) splenius capitis; (c) temporalis; (d) masseter; (e) trapezius; (f) levator scapulae; (g) posterior cervical; (h) infraspinatus; (i) supraspinatus; (j) middle finger extensor; (k) extensor carpi radialis; (l) supinators; (m) pectoralis minor; (n) pectoralis major; (o) sternalis; (p) gluteus medius; (q) iliocostalis lumborum; (r) serratus anterior; (s) multifidi and rotatores; (t) gluteus minimus; (u) vastus medialis; (v) abductor hallucis; (w) short extensors

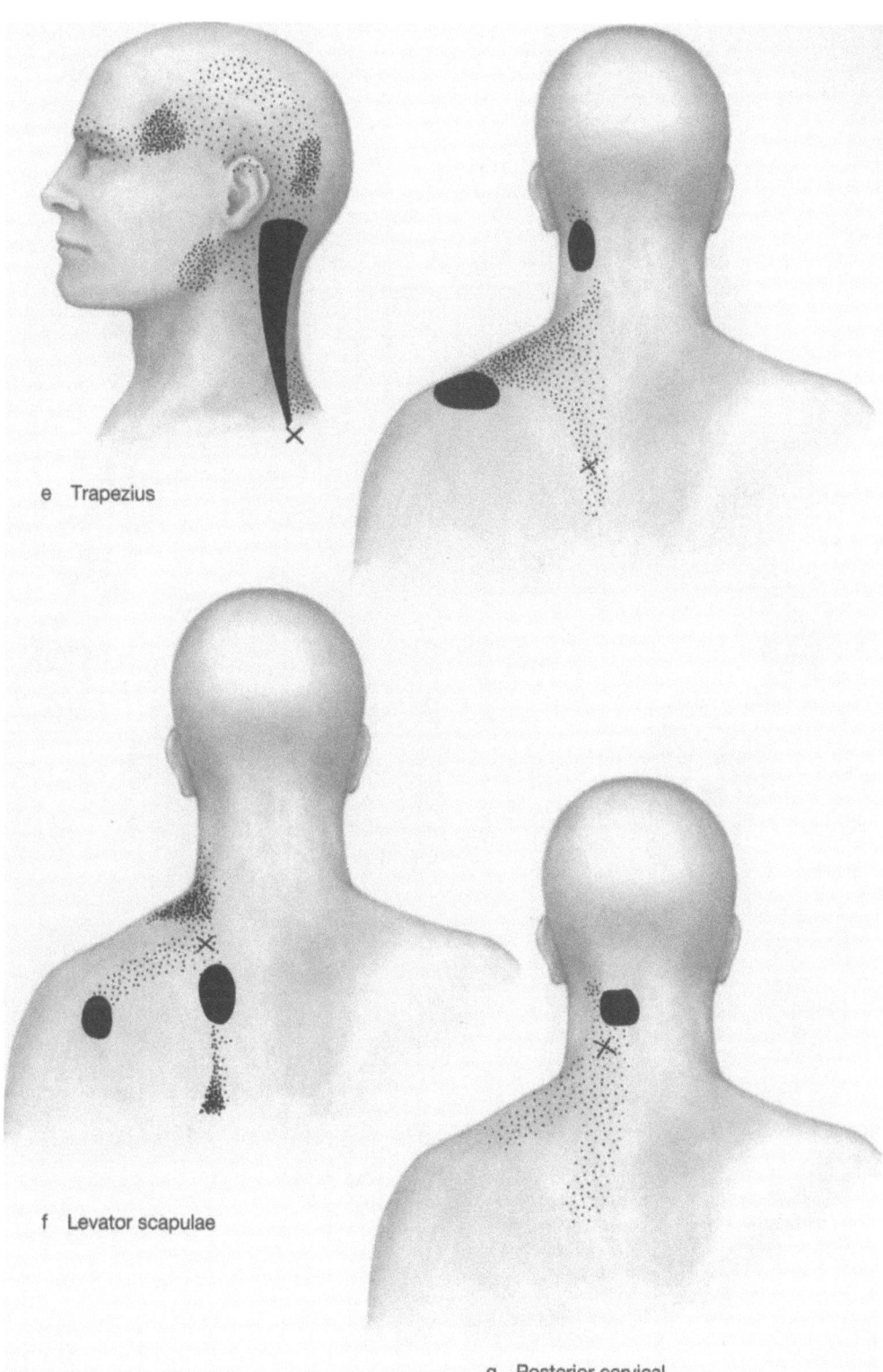

e   Trapezius

f   Levator scapulae

g   Posterior cervical

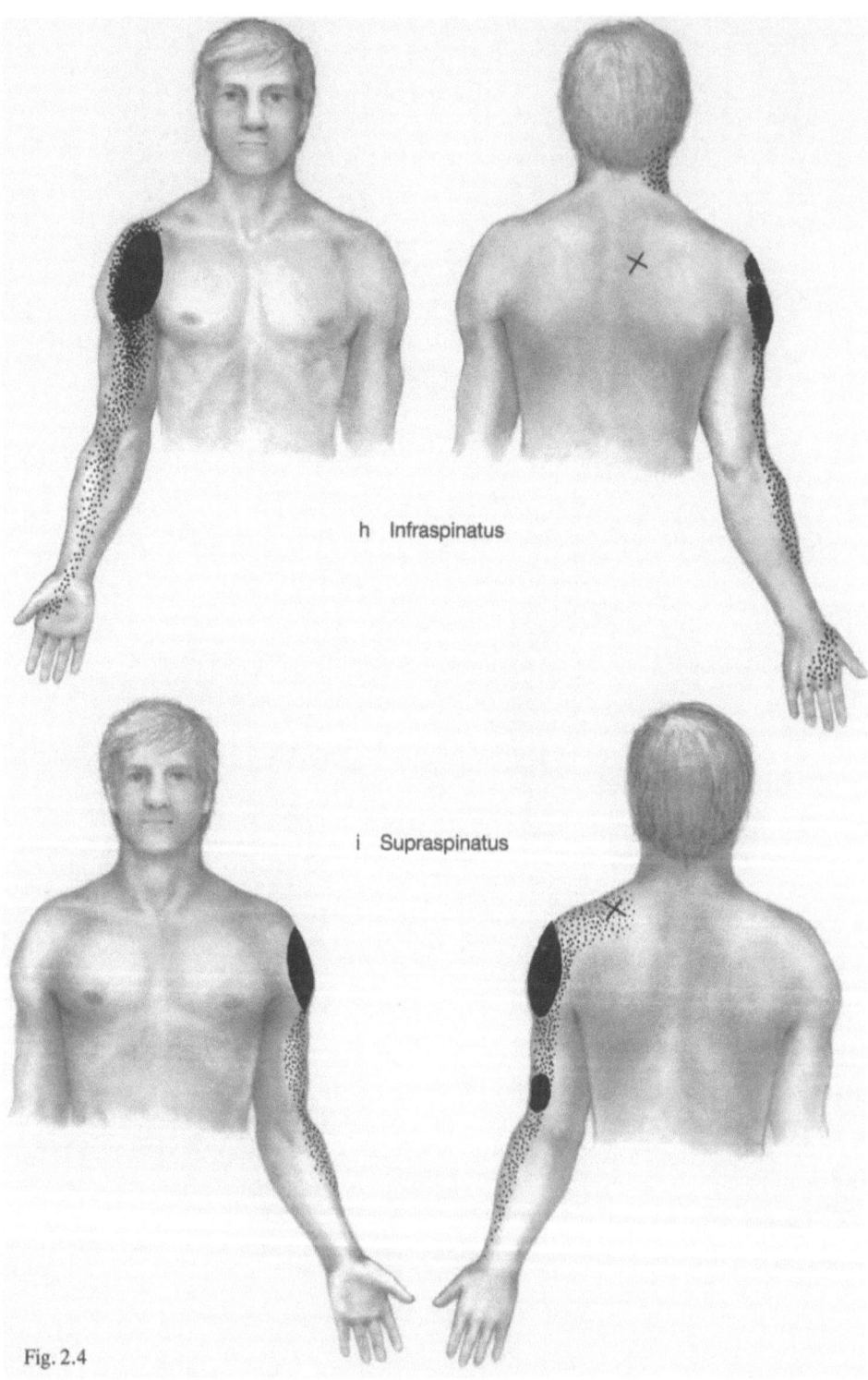

h   Infraspinatus

i   Supraspinatus

Fig. 2.4

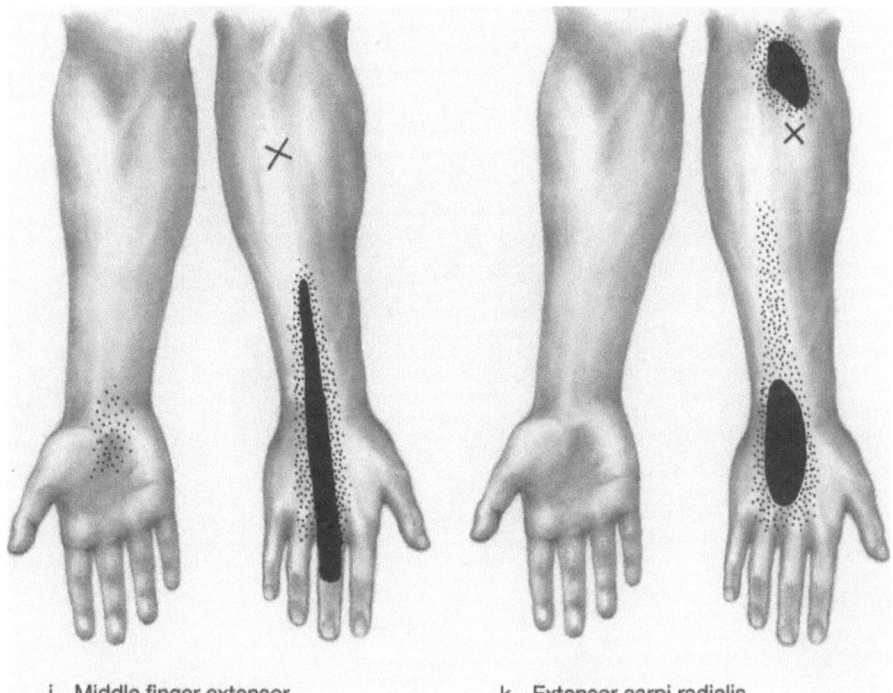

j  Middle finger extensor          k  Extensor carpi radialis

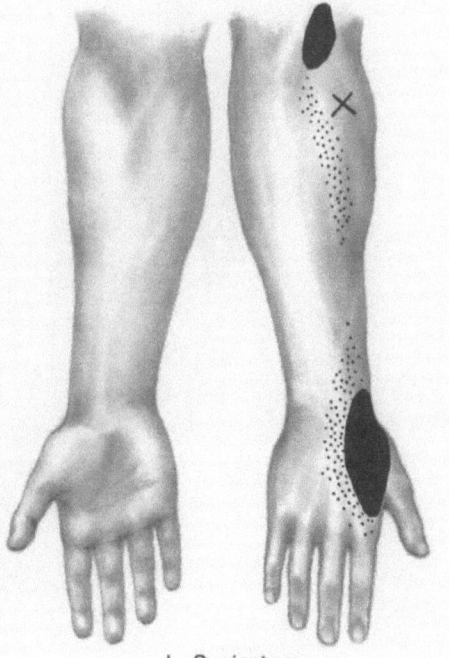

Fig. 2.4                              l  Supinators

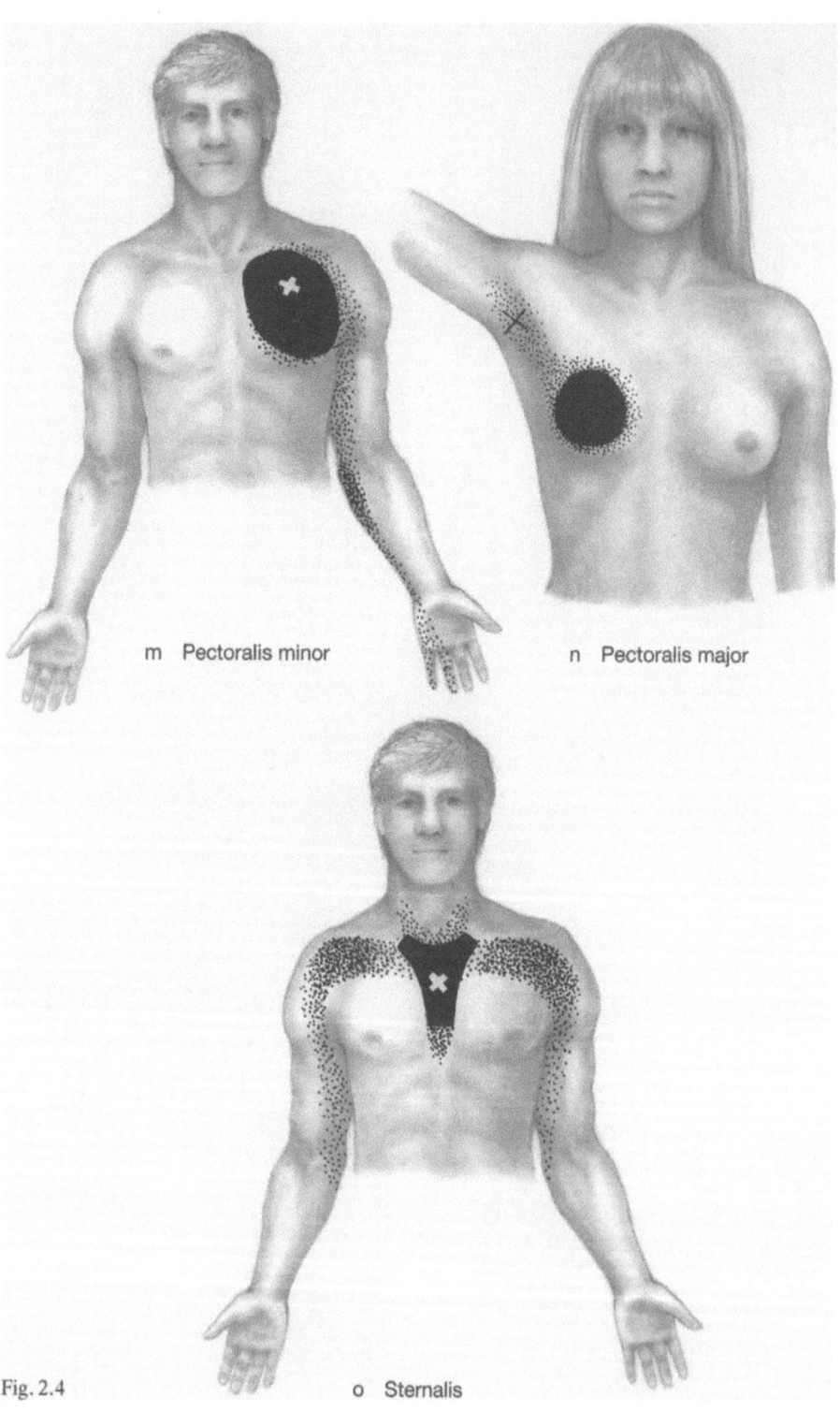

m Pectoralis minor      n Pectoralis major

Fig. 2.4         o Sternalis

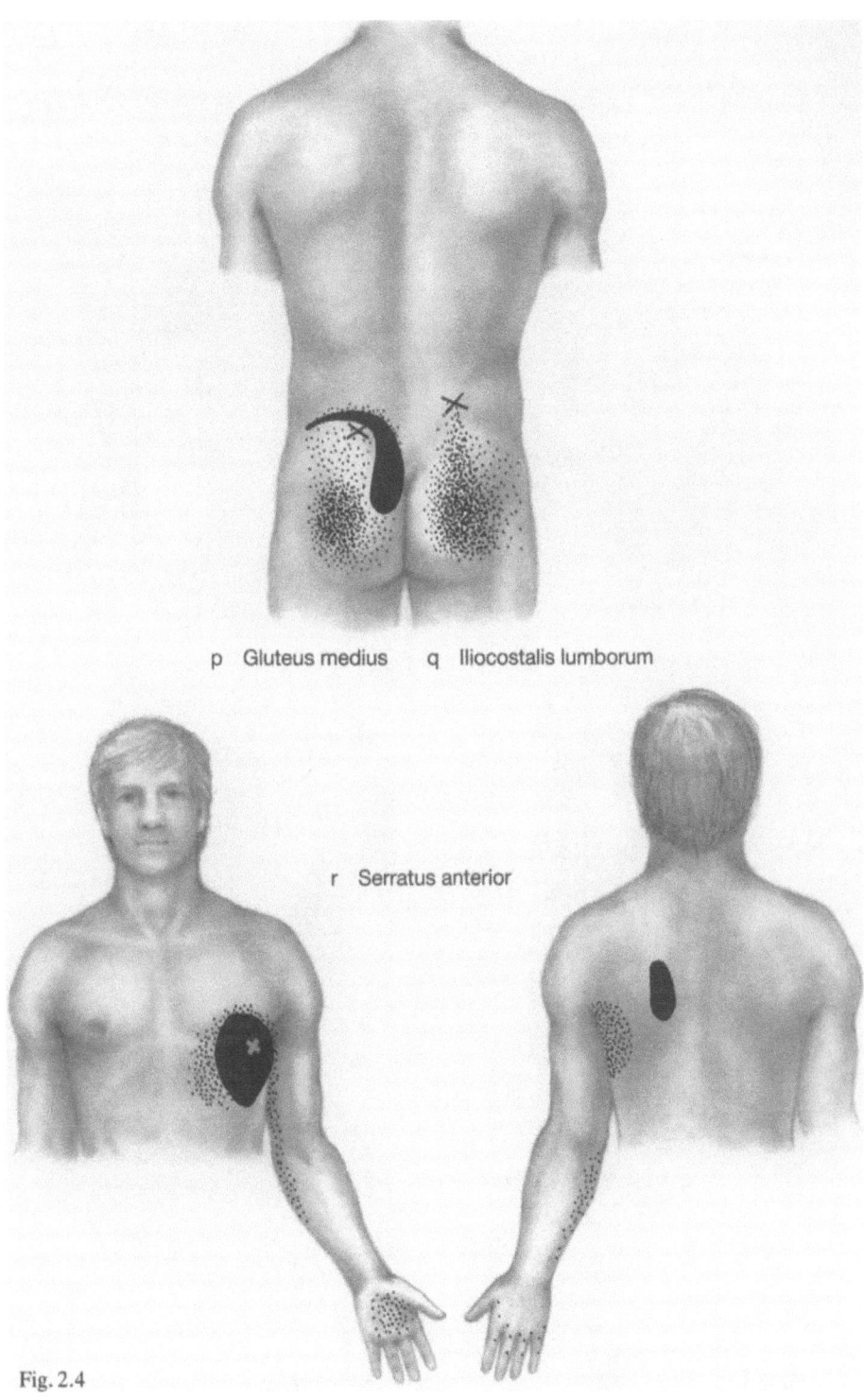

p   Gluteus medius    q   Iliocostalis lumborum

r   Serratus anterior

Fig. 2.4

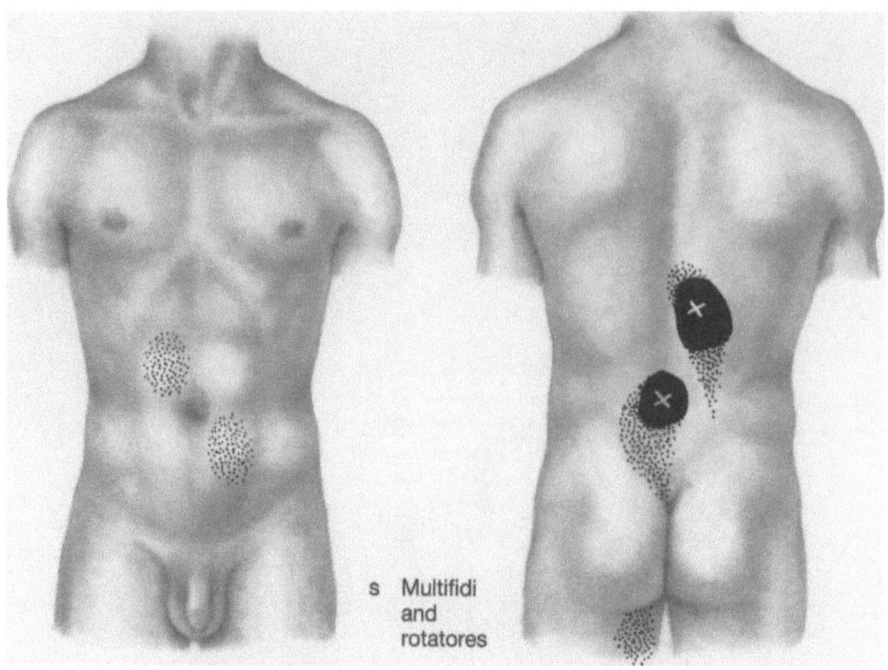

s  Multifidi
   and
   rotatores

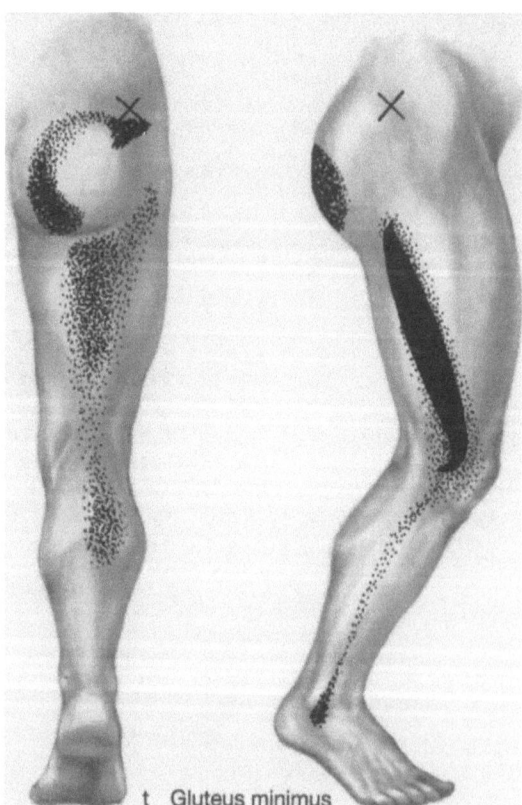

Fig. 2.4

t  Gluteus minimus

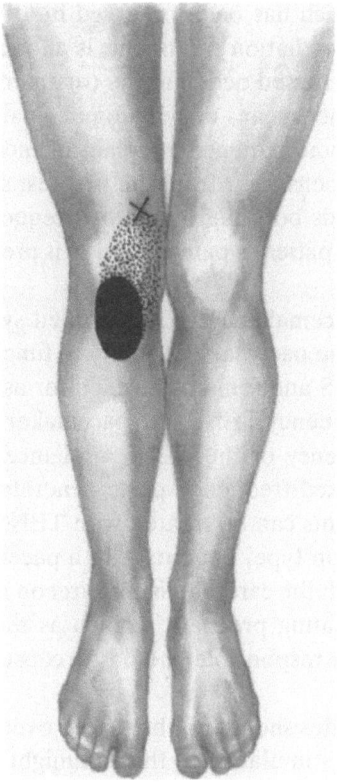

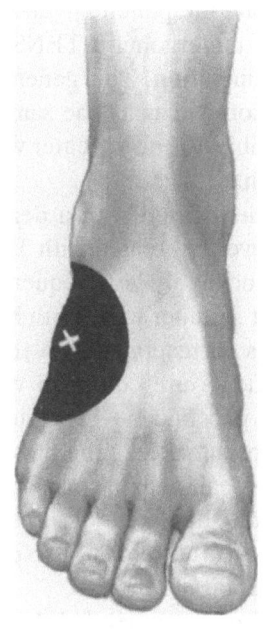

u   Vastus medialis

v   Abductor hallucis

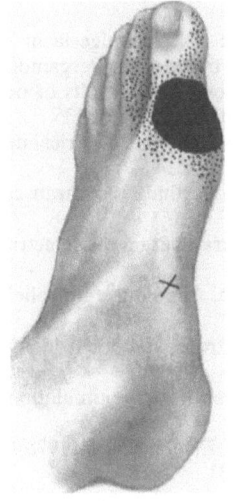

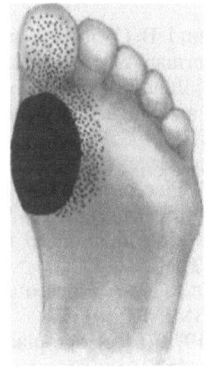

w   Short extensors

Fig. 2.4

A further side effect of TENS, which has been observed in a few patients who have undergone mastectomy and radiation treatment, is an increased tendency to oedema. If TENS leads to increased oedema, the treatment should be stopped and the patient given some other means of symptomatic pain relief.

When undergoing a TENS test, some patients complain of increased pain during stimulation. This generally happens right from the first test session, and the reaction is usually the same towards both high- and low-frequency TENS. This possibility is also greater when the patient's pain condition is predominantly psychogenic.

A patient fitted with a demand pacemaker (ECG-controlled synchronous) should never be treated with TENS. The pacemaker's ability to function is completely blocked by low-frequency TENS and remains blocked for as long as the treatment is under way. With high-frequency TENS, the pacemaker may generate pulses corresponding to the frequency of the TENS appliance. However, some patients are equipped with a fixed-frequency pulse generator − a synchronous pacemaker − and such patients can be treated with TENS. Since the demand pacemaker is the most common type, patients with a pacemaker must always be dealt with in consultation with the cardiologist or surgeon responsible.

Caution should be observed in treating pregnant women as there may be some risk to the foetus. The physician responsible should be consulted before treatment starts.

It is also recommended that electrodes should not be placed over the carotid arteries as there is a potential risk that stimulation at this site might cause heart block by exciting the vagus nerve.

## References

Eriksson M, Sjölund B (1976) Acupuncture-like electroanalgesia in TNS-resistant chronic pain. In: Zotterman Y (ed) Sensory functions of the skin. Pergamon Press, Oxford, p 575

Eriksson MBE, Sjölund BH, Nielzén S (1979) Long term results of peripheral conditioning stimulation as an analgesic measure in chronic pain. Pain 6:335

Gersh MR, Woolf SL (1985) Applications of transcutaneous electrical nerve stimulation in the management of patients with pain. Phys Ther 85:314

Laitinen L (1976) Placement d'électrodes dans la stimulation transcutanée de la douleur chronique. Neurochirurgie 22:517

Lampe GN (1978) Introduction to the use of transcutaneous electrical nerve stimulation devices. Phys Ther 58:1450

Linzer M, Long DM (1976) Transcutaneous neural stimulation for relief of pain. IEEE Trans Biomed Eng BME-23:341

Mannheimer JS (1978) Electrode placements for transcutaneous electrical nerve stimulation. Phys Ther 58:1455

Pomeranz B (1987) Antinociception from peripheral nerve stimulation in rats and humans. Pain [Suppl] 4:S679

Thorsteinsson G, Stonnington HH, Stillwell GK, Elveback LR (1978) The placebo effect of transcutaneous electrical stimulation. Pain 5:31

Travell J, Rinzler SH (1952) Myofascial genesis of pain. Postgrad Med J 11:425

Travell J, Simmons D (1983) Myofascial pain and dysfunction. The trigger point manual. William and Wilkins, Baltimore

Wall PD, Melzack R (eds) (1984) Textbook of pain. Churchill Livingstone, Edinburgh
Wall PD, Sweet WH (1967) Temporary abolition of pain in man. Science 155:108
Wang K, Yao S, Xian Y, Hou Z (1985) A study on the receptive field of acupoints and the relationship between characteristics of needle sensation and groups of afferent fibres. Sci Sin [B] 28:963
Woolf CJ (1984) Transcutaneous and implanted nerve stimulation. In: Wall PD, Melzack R (eds) Textbook of pain. Churchill Livingstone, Edinburgh, p 679
Woolf SL, Gersh MR, Rao VR (1981) Examination of electrode placements and stimulating parameters in treating chronic pain with conventional transcutaneous electrical nerve stimulation (TENS). Pain 11:37

## Suggested Reading

Andersson SA, Erikson T, Holmgren E, Lindqvist G (1973) Electroacupuncture. Effect on pain threshold measured with electrical stimulation of teeth. Brain Res 63:393
Andersson SA, Holmgren E (1976) Pain threshold effects of peripheral conditioning stimulation. In: Bonica JJ, Albe-Fessard (eds) Advances in pain research and therapy, vol 1. Raven, New York, p 761
Colwell HA (1922) An essay on the history of electrotherapy and diagnosis. Heinemann, London
Dalziel DF, Lee WR (1969) Lethal and electric current. IEEE Spectrum 6:44
Eriksson M, Schuller H, Sjölund B (1978) Hazard from transcutaneous nerve stimulation in patients with pacemakers. Lancet 1:1319
Geddes LA, Cabler P, Moore AG, Rosborough J, Tacker WA (1973) Threshold 60 Hz current required for ventricular fibrillation in subjects of various body weights. IEEE Trans Biomed Eng BMW-20:465
Kane K, Taub A (1975) A history of local electrical analgesia. Pain 1:125
Kellaway P (1946) The part played by electric fish in the early history of bioelectricity and electrotherapy. Bull Hist Med 20:112
Mason CP (1976) Testing of electrical transcutaneous stimulators for suppressing pain. Bull Prosthetics Res, Spring:38
Picaza IA, Cannon BW, Hunter SE, Boyd AS, Guma J, Maurer D (1975) Pain suppression by peripheral nerve stimulation. I. Observations with transcutaneous stimuli. Surg Neurol 4:105
Schecter DC (1971) Origins of electrotherapy. NY State J Med 71:997
Veale JL, Mark RF, Rees S (1973) Differential sensitivity of motor and sensory fibres in human ulnar nerve. J Neurol Neurosurg Psychiatry 36:75
Zugermann C (1982) Dermatitis from transcutaneous electric nerve stimulation. J Am Acad Dermatol 6:936

# *Chapter 3*   TENS in Different Pain Syndromes

## Post-operative Pain

In recent decades a large number of reports have been published concerning post-operative pain and its alleviation. Analgesic drugs may produce unwanted side effects and prolong the time of rehabilitation after surgery. The use of peripheral stimulation for the alleviation of post-operative pain may prove to be an alternative.

### Usefulness of TENS in Post-operative Pain

One of the most successful applications of TENS is for post-operative pain control. There is evidence from recent studies that TENS not only reduces post-operative pain, but also the incidence of complications such as paralytic ileus and atelectasis and may increase the mobility of the patient and shorten the recovery period.

Before surgery the patient should be informed about the potential benefits of TENS and instructed in the use of the apparatus. Post-operatively TENS treatment should start in the recovery room, and stimulation be continuous for the first 2 h. After this time the effects of anaesthesia have subsided sufficiently, and the patient is generally able to describe any post-operative pain and his perception of the TENS stimulation. The clinician may then have to re-adjust the intensity controls to obtain the optimal effect. The patient should not manipulate the controls at this stage. Stimulation may be continuous or at intervals, such as 2 h on, 2 h off. For the 1st day the electrodes should remain in place. If sterile long-lasting electrodes are used, they may be kept in place for up to 3 days. The electrode site should be checked daily for the presence of skin irritation, adequate electrode contact and continuity of adhesive tape. Faulty electrodes should be replaced, and inadequate electrode placement rectified.

Three days of intermittent or continuous stimulation is sufficient in most post-operative cases. Additional stimulation may be required in difficult cases, and some patients may require the use of a TENS apparatus on a home programme. The patient will require in-depth instruction on how to maintain and adjust the unit.

Several investigators have studied the efficacy of TENS for management of post-operative pain. In many of these studies, electrodes were placed parallel to

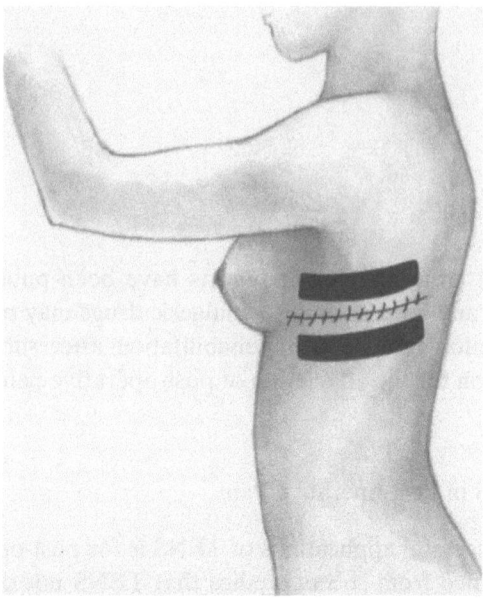

Fig. 3.1. Post-thoracotomy incision pain. *Electrode placement sites:* on both sides of incision. *Recommended mode of stimulation:* high frequency, intensity just below pain threshold. *Polarity:* generally of no importance

the incision, stimulation set at comfortable levels, and TENS used for hours continuously for at least the first 24–48 h. The treatment was discontinued after that period at each patient's request. All investigators reported a significant decrease in the dosages of pain medication requested by the patients using TENS compared with those patients not using TENS (Vander Ark and McGrath 1975; Navaratham et al. 1984; Pike 1978; Schomburg and Carter-Baker 1983; Solomon et al. 1980; Jensen et al. 1985). Furthermore, several authors have reported rehabilitation benefits when using TENS to control post-operative pain (Harvie 1979; Arvidsson and Eriksson 1986; Schuster and Infante 1980; Stabile and Mallory 1978). However, some authors (Gilbert et al. 1986; Conn et al. 1986) claim that TENS is no better than placebo in alleviating post-operative pain.

Patients with pulmonary disease seem to respond well to treatment with TENS and, in particular, those with asthma and emphysema may find it helps improve their breathing. TENS may be used along with measures such as breathing exercises, relaxation and upper extremity mobilisation. Patients receiving physical or inhalation therapy may derive benefit from the reduction of chest pain by the application of TENS for 1–2 h, twice daily, allowing improved respiration and increased vital capacity.

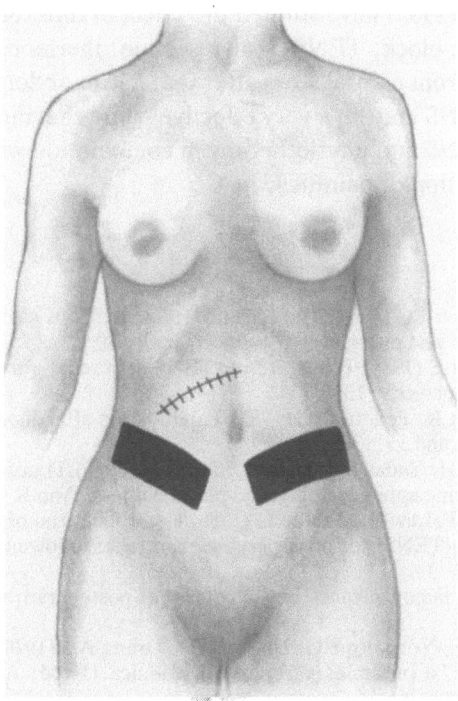

Fig. 3.2. Post-operative ileus pain. *Electrode placement sites:* on the abdomen above the ascending and descending colon. *Recommended mode of stimulation:* high frequency, intensity just below pain threshold. *Polarity:* generally of no importance

Ali et al. (1981) studied the pulmonary function of 40 patients who had undergone cholecystectomies. Fifteen patients used TENS continuously for the first 48 h post-operatively and then on an "as needed" basis. Another 15 patients who served as controls did not use TENS, and a third group of ten patients used TENS units with the batteries reversed so that no current was delivered to the patient (sham TENS). Spirometric evaluations of all patients, conducted on the 3rd and 5th post-operative days, indicated that patients who were treated with TENS had significantly higher vital capacities and functional residual capacities than patients receiving either sham TENS or no TENS. Patients using TENS had a significantly decreased incidence of post-operative pulmonary dysfunction and complications. Patients in all groups required supplemental pain medications, but those in the TENS group required less than those not receiving actual TENS treatment.

The effects of TENS on paralytic ileus and atelectasis after abdominal surgery have been examined by Hymes et al. (1974a, b). They have shown that 13% of the TENS group of patients having undergone abdominal surgery developed atelectasis compared to 27% of the control group.

Carlsson et al. (1985) have studied the effect of different treatment methods including analgesic block, TENS, scar resection, thermocoagulation, etc. in 37 patients suffering from painful scars after thoracic or abdominal surgery. The results show that TENS may be a very effective pain-relieving measure and the authors advocate TENS and physiotherapy in combination with psychological support for the alleviation of painful scars.

## References

Ali JA, Yaffe CS, Seretti C (1981) The effect of transcutaneous electric nerve stimulation on postoperative pain and pulmonary function. Surgery 89:507

Arvidsson J, Eriksson E (1986) Postoperative TENS pain relief after knee surgery: objective evaluation. Orthopedics 9:1346

Carlsson CA, Persson K, Pelletieri L (1985) Painful scars after thoracic and abdominal surgery. Acta Chir Scand 151:309

Conn JG, Marshall AH, Yadav SN, Daly JC, Jaffer M (1986) Transcutaneous electrical nerve stimulation following appendectomy: the placebo effect. Ann R Coll Surg Engl 68:191

Gilbert JM, Gledhill T, Law N, George C (1986) Controlled trial of transcutaneous electrical nerve stimulation (TENS) for postoperative pain relief following inguinal herniorrhaphy. Br J Surg 73:749

Harvie KW (1979) A major advance in the control of postoperative knee pain. Orthopedics 2:1

Hymes AC, Raab DE, Yonchiro EG, Nelson GD, Drintz AL (1974a) Acute pain control by electrostimulation: a preliminary report. In: Bonica JJ (ed) Advances in neurology 4. Raven, New York, p 761

Hymes AC, Yonehiro EG, Raab DE, Nelson GD, Drintz AL (1974b) Electrical surface stimulation for treatment and prevention of ileus and atelectasis. Surg Forum 25:222

Jensen JE, Conn RR, Hazelrigg G, Hewett JE (1985) The use of transcutaneous neural stimulation and isokinetic testing in arthroscopic knee surgery. Am J Sports Med 13:27

Navaratham RG, Wang IY, Thomas D, Kineberg PL (1984) Evaluation of the transcutaneous electrical nerve stimulator for postoperative analgesia following cardiac surgery. Anaesth Intensive Care 12:345

Pike PMH (1978) Transcutaneous electrical stimulation: its use in the management of postoperative pain. Anaesthesia 33:165

Schomburg FL, Carter-Baker SA (1983) Transcutaneous electrical nerve stimulation for post-laparatomy pain. Phys Ther 63:188

Schuster GD, Infante MC (1980) Pain relief after low back surgery: the efficacy of TENS. Pain 8:299

Solomon RA, Viernstein MC, Long DM (1980) Reduction of postoperative pain and narcotic use by transcutaneous electrical nerve stimulation. Surgery 87:142

Stabile ML, Mallory TH (1978) The management of postoperative pain in total joint replacement: transcutaneous electrical nerve stimulation is evaluated in total hip and knee patients. Ortho Rev 7:121

Vander Ark GD, McGrath KA (1975) Transcutaneous electrical stimulation in treatment of postoperative pain. Am J Surg 130:338

## Suggested Reading

Cooperman AM, Hall B, Mikalacki K, Hardy R, Sadar E (1977) Use of transcutaneous electrical stimulation in control of postoperative pain – results of prospective, randomized, controlled study. Am J Surg 133:185

Rosenberg M, Curtis L, Bourke DL (1978) Transcutaneous electric nerve stimulation for the relief of postoperative pain. Pain 5:129

# Neck and Shoulder Pain

Pain from the shoulder and neck can be placed in the following categories: (a) pain primarily in the neck; (b) neck-shoulder pain; and (c) pain primarily in the shoulders. Physical examination of the patient who presents with any of these complaints must include the neck, the root of the neck, the scapular and inter-scapular areas, pectoral regions, the clavicles and the axilla.

Localised neck or suboccipital pain is mediated through the branches of the posterior primary rami of the spinal nerves and cervical plexus. The neck-shoulder pain is also mediated through the posterior spinal nerve branches. Localised shoulder pain is mediated through the branches of the brachial plexus to the shoulder joint. The shoulder plus radiating pain symptoms are from nerve root injury or due to vascular irritation and are mediated through various pathways.

One of the most common causes of acute neck or shoulder pain is cervical strain. Cervical strain is a derangement of the sternocleidomastoid musculo-tendonous junction at the mastoid process and results in increased tone in the sternocleidomastoid muscle. The pain may be perceived behind the ear. Charac-teristically, the pain is not related to rotation, and the aching is more lateral than the discomfort noted in suboccipital arthritis. However, the tenderness is often unilateral and extends over the mastoid process. Patients with chronic strain have usually had a whiplash injury, i.e. an extension-flexion injury to the cervi-cal spine. Apart from whiplash injuries, car accidents may result in lesions of the brachial plexus causing severe long-lasting cervical pain. Generally these lesions are very resistant to therapy.

Arthritis of the cervical spine can be considered a normal development of middle age. It is important to note that even if patients have degenerative changes in the cervical spine at X-ray examination, they may not have any symptoms al-though strain trauma or debilitating disease may trigger off the pain. Other types of degenerative conditions of the spine such as rheumatoid arthritis may also cause symptoms in the cervico-occipital region. In patients with arthritic changes in the cervical spine, the pain is primarily induced by neck motion and may ex-tend into the shoulder or present with headaches. It is usually associated with stiffness which increases during the day.

The neck and the neck-shoulder pain is usually described as aching or gnaw-ing in character. It is often difficult for these patients to localise their pain which may be described as diffuse. Sometimes the pain is sharp or gripping, and it can produce tingling. Associated conditions such as fibrositis, scapulothoracic dis-orders, neurological and postural disturbances resulting from strain of the erector muscles are not uncommon, as are also round shoulders and pendulous breasts. The complaint is often bilateral.

The shoulder plus radiating pain pattern may be caused by extruded and de-generative discs as well as foraminal compression and spondylotic changes − the cervical root syndrome. Degenerated discs cause local pain in the neck plus radiating pain to the arm. Pain may increase when the head is tilted towards the side of the disc protrusion and decrease when tilted to the other side. These patients have intermittent bouts of discomfort that are relieved by rest, by the use of a cervical collar, hot packs, massage, trigger point injections, analgesics, anti-inflammatory medications, muscle relaxants or other conservative treatment.

Cord tumor and fractures form a small percentage of root syndrome problems. The pain radiates from the neck distally, often a sharp and shooting pain aggravated by coughing, sneezing and neck movement. The pain pattern is usually fairly specific along dermatomal patterns.

## Usefulness of TENS in Neck and Shoulder Pain

Nordemar and Thörner (1981) randomised 30 patients with acute cervical pain due to cervical strain into three treatment groups; neck collar, high-frequency TENS and manual therapy. The improvement was rapid in all groups but the restoration of cervical mobility was significantly more rapid in the TENS group. Parry (1980) reported that 50% of patients with avulsion injuries of the brachial plexus obtained significant relief with high-frequency TENS. The most effective electrode placement sites were centrally at the C5-C7 levels and just proximal to the site of pain where afferent input was still present. The patients for whom TENS was not beneficial had total lesions of the plexus. Parry states that TENS should be used for at least 2 h at a time, two to three times a day and sometimes for up to 6–8 h. In a long-term follow-up of 108 patients with avulsion lesions, Parry showed that drugs are of very limited use, and the most valuable method of treatment found was TENS although only one-third responded dramatically to this treatment.

Reports by Shealy (1974), Crue and Felsoory (1974) and Mannheimer and Lampe (1984) show that TENS can be used for the alleviation of arthritis of the cervical spine and neck-shoulder discomfort. Generally, the best effects have resulted from placing the electrodes suboccipitally or over the transverse process of C2 bilaterally. Kaada (1984) has reported that TENS can be used in patients suffering from calcareous shoulder. Out of 14 patients treated, two were classified as acute, nine as chronic, and three as asymptomatic. Significant relief of pain and increased mobility were obtained in ten of the 11 patients 1–2 weeks after daily stimulation was commenced.

Mannheimer and Lampe (1984) have reported that TENS can be very effective in the modulation of shoulder pain due to musculoskeletal dysfunction. According to them, TENS should be used in the acute phase (tendinitis or bursitis) as a symptomatic treatment along with joint mobilisation to maintain laxity of the capsule and prevent loss of movement. These procedures should prevent the development of a periarthritis and ensuing chronic pain.

## References

Crue BL Jr, Felsoory A (1974) Transcutaneous high cervical "electrical cordotomy". Minn Med J 57:204

Kaada B (1984) Treatment of peritendinitis calcarea of the shoulder by transcutaneous nerve stimulation. Acupunct Electrother Res 9:115

Mannheimer JS, Lampe GN (1984) Clinical transcutaneous electrical nerve stimulation. Davis, Philadelphia

Nordemar R, Thörner C (1981) Treatment of acute cervical pain — a comparative study group. Pain 10:93

Parry CBW (1980) Pain in avulsion lesions of the brachial plexus. Pain 9:41

Shealy CN (1974) Electrical control of the nervous system. Med Prog Technol 2:71

## Suggested Reading

Cauthen JC, Renner EJ (1975) Transcutaneous and peripheral nerve stimulation for chronic pain states. Surg Neurol 4:102

Lampe GN (1977) A clinical approach to transcutaneous electrical nerve stimulation in the treatment of acute and chronic pain. Medgeneral, Minneapolis, p 31

Long DM (1973) Electrical stimulation for relief of pain from chronic nerve injury. J Neurosurg 39:718

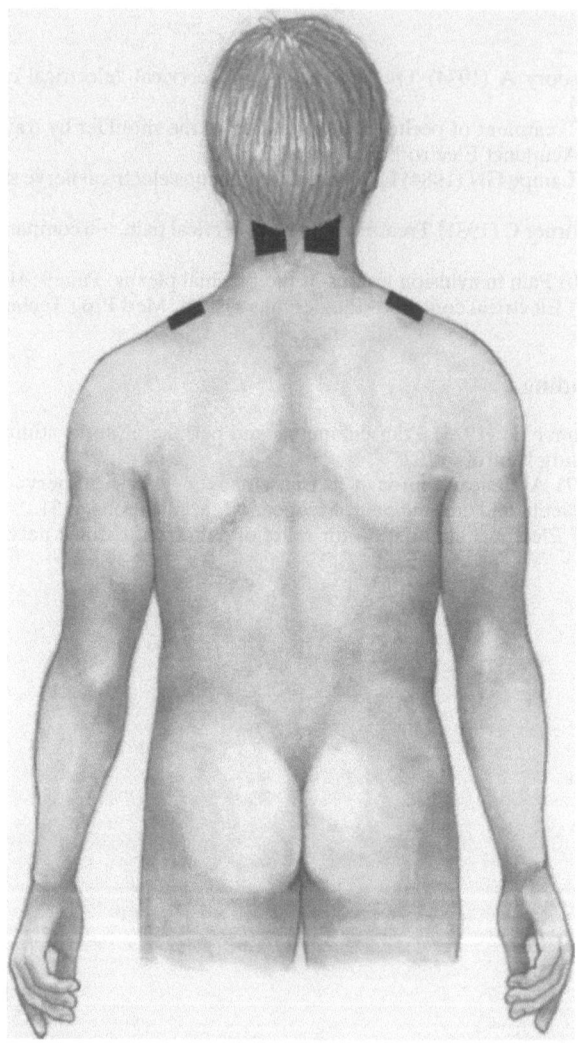

Fig. 3.3. Cervical strain — acute. *Electrode placement sites:* suboccipital fossa bilaterally and upper trapezius bilaterally. *Recommended mode of stimulation:* high frequency or low-frequency trains, intensity just below pain threshold. *Polarity:* generally of no importance

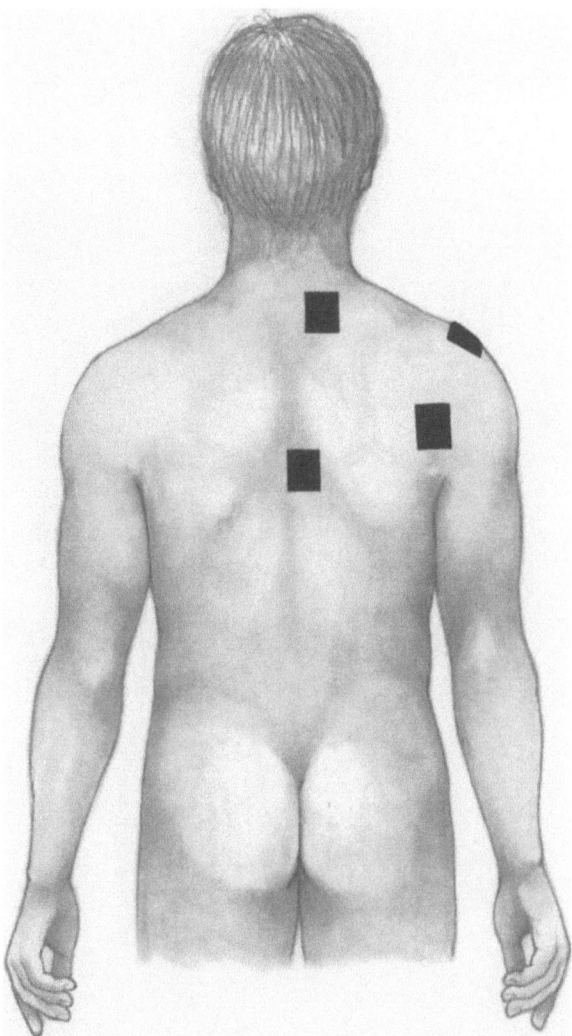

Fig. 3.4. Cervical strain – acute. *Electrode placement sites:* one pair at posterior axillary fold and cervicothoracic junction; another pair at musculotendinous junction of supraspinatus and paraspinal at T6–7. *Recommended mode of stimulation:* high frequency or low-frequency trains, intensity just below pain threshold. *Polarity:* generally of no importance

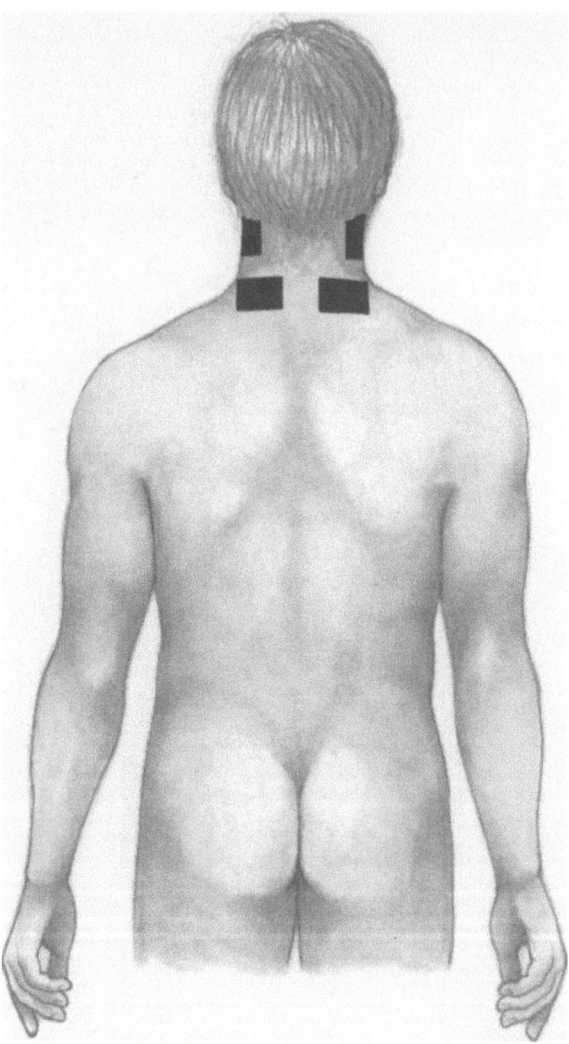

Fig. 3.5. Cervical strain – chronic. *Electrode placement sites:* one pair bilaterally at suboccipital fossa and another pair at cervicothoracic junction paravertebrally. *Recommended mode of stimulation:* high frequency or low-frequency trains, intensity just below pain threshold. *Polarity:* generally of no importance

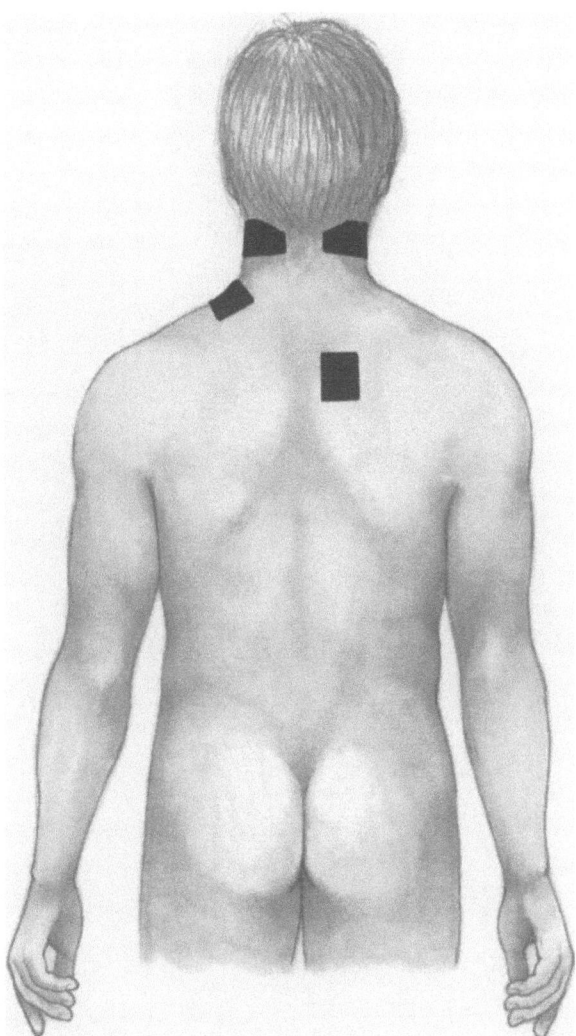

Fig. 3.6. Cervical spine pain. *Electrode placement sites:* one pair at suboccipital fossa bilateral-ly: another pair just below spine of scapula on vertebral border and just inferior to upper trapezius motor/trigger point. *Recommended mode of stimulation:* high frequency or low-fre-quency trains, intensity just below pain threshold. *Polarity:* generally of no importance

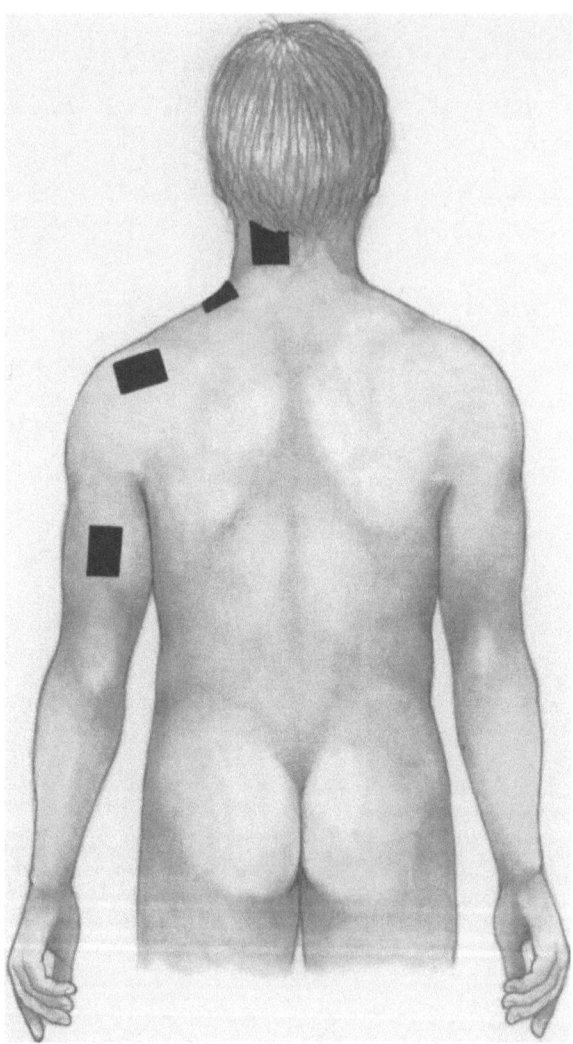

Fig. 3.7. Cervical spine pain. *Electrode placement sites:* one pair paravertebrally at C3–C5 and upper trapezius; another pair in depression below posterior aspect of acromion and posterior aspect of arm just above elbow. *Recommended mode of stimulation:* high frequency or low-frequency trains, intensity just below pain threshold. *Polarity:* generally of no importance

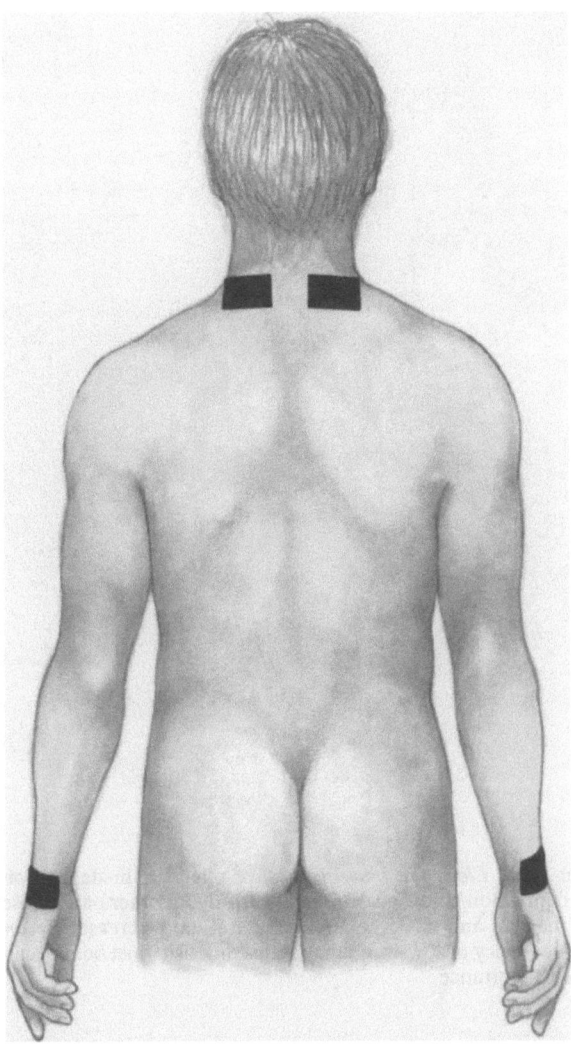

Fig. 3.8. Cervical spine pain. *Electrode placement sites:* cervicothoracic junction and overlying flexor carpi ulnaris on both left and right side. *Recommended mode of stimulation:* brief, intense low-frequency TENS (producing rhythmical contractions. *Polarity:* generally of no importance

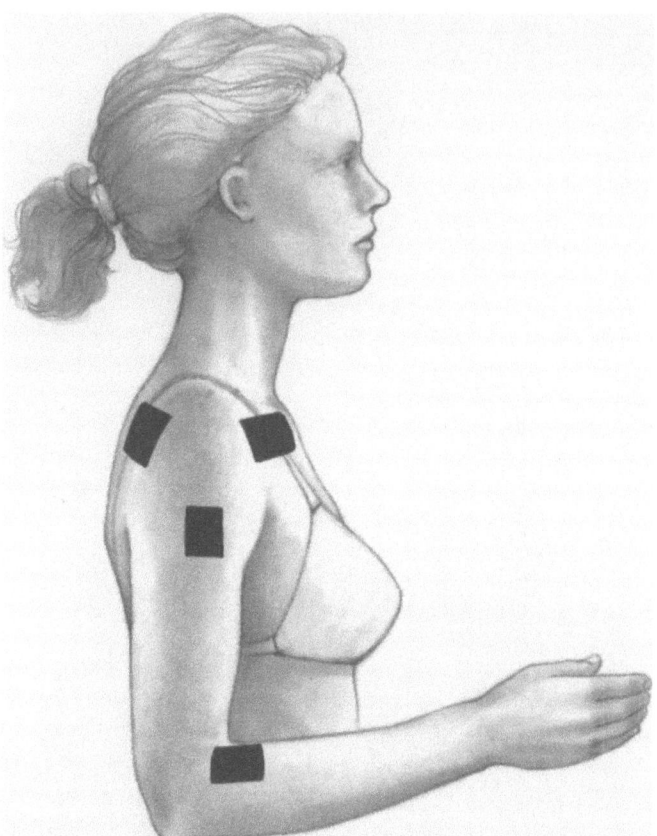

Fig. 3.9. Shoulder pain. *Electrode placement sites:* one pair in depression below acromion anteriorly and in depression below acromion posteriorly; another pair at insertion of deltoid at lateral aspect of the arm and in depression of lateral elbow crease. *Recommended mode of stimulation:* high frequency or low-frequency trains, intensity just below pain threshold. *Polarity:* generally of no importance

Fig. 3.10. Shoulder pain. *Electrode placement sites:* one pair in depression below acromion anteriorly and in depression below acromion posteriorly; another pair in depression bordered by the acromion, scapula and clavicle and at insertion of deltoid at lateral aspect of arm. *Recommended mode of stimulation:* high frequency or low-frequency trains, intensity just below pain threshold. *Polarity:* generally of no importance

Fig. 3.11. Shoulder pain. *Electrode placement sites:* one pair in depression below acromion anteriorly and in depression below acromion posteriorly; another pair at insertion of deltoid at lateral aspect of arm and dorsal web space. *Recommended mode of stimulation:* high frequency or low-frequency trains, intensity just below pain threshold. *Polarity:* generally of no importance

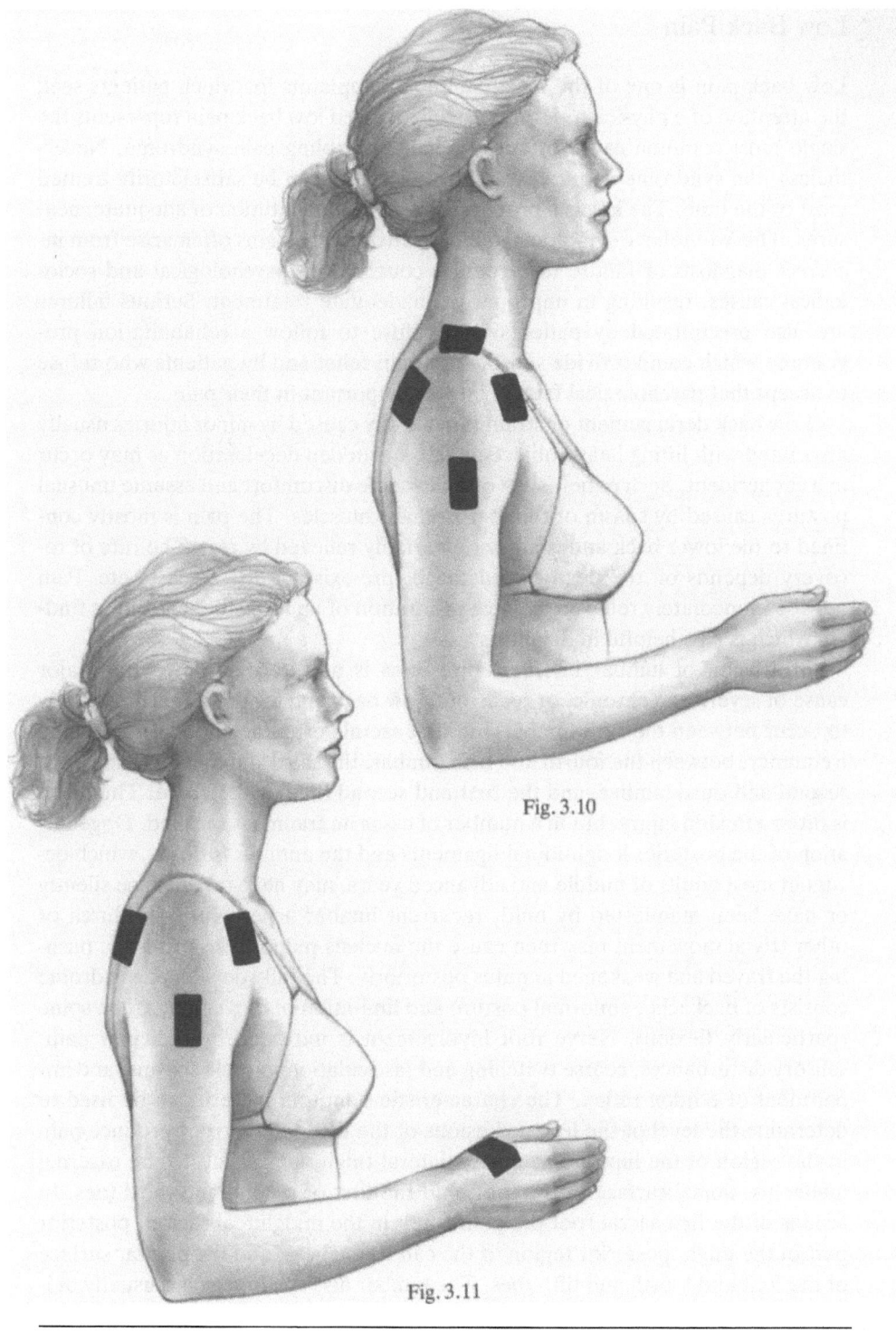

Fig. 3.10

Fig. 3.11

## Low Back Pain

Low back pain is one of the most common complaints for which patients seek the attention of a physician. Unsuccessfully treated low back pain represents the single most common cause of an intractable disabling pain syndrome. Nevertheless, the syndrome is quite straightforward and can be satisfactorily treated most of the time. The key is a proper diagnosis and institution of adequate measures. This will relieve symptoms in most patients. Problems often arise from incorrect diagnosis or failure to recognise concomitant psychological and sociological causes, resulting in improper or inadequate treatment. Serious failures are also precipitated by patients who refuse to follow a rehabilitation programme which could provide satisfactory pain relief and by patients who refuse to accept that psychological factors may be important in their pain.

Low back derangement or strain is generally caused by minor injuries usually associated with lifting heavy objects, a fall, or sudden deceleration as may occur in a car accident. Such patients are often in acute discomfort and assume unusual postures caused by spasm of the sacrospinalis muscles. The pain is mostly confined to the lower back and is almost invariably relieved by rest. The rate of recovery depends on the degree of damage, pre-existing disc disease, etc. Pain may be immediately relieved by local infiltration of an anaesthetic agent, a finding which is also helpful in diagnosis.

Protrusion of lumbar intervertebral discs is now recognised as the major cause of severe and chronic, or recurrent, low back and leg pain. It is most likely to occur between the fifth lumbar and first sacral vertebrae and, with lessening frequency, between the fourth and fifth lumbar, the third and fourth lumbar, the second and third lumbar, and the first and second lumbar vertebrae. The cause is often a flexion injury, but in a number of cases no trauma is recalled. Degeneration of the posterior longitudinal ligaments and the annulus fibrosus, which occurs in most adults of middle and advanced years, may have taken place silently or have been manifested by mild, recurrent lumbar ache. A sneeze, lurch or other trivial movement may then cause the nucleus pulposus to prolapse, pushing the frayed and weakened annulus posteriorly. The fully developed syndrome consists of backache, abnormal posture and limitation of movement of the spine (particularly flexion). Nerve root involvement is indicated by radicular pain, sensory disturbances, coarse twitching and fasciculation, muscle spasms, and impairment of tendon reflex. The characteristic symptom pattern can be used to determine the level of the lesion. Lesions of the fifth lumbar root produce pain in the region of the hip, groin, posterolateral thigh, lateral calf to the external malleolus, dorsal surface of the foot, and the first or second and third toes. In lesions of the first sacral root the pain is felt in the midgluteal region, posterior part of the thigh, posterior region of the calf to the heel, and the plantar surface of the foot and fourth and fifth toes. The lumbar disc syndromes are usually unilateral. The pain may be mild to severe. There may be back pain with little or no leg pain; rarely, only leg pain may be experienced. The rupture of multiple lumbar or lumbar and cervical discs is not infrequent.

Arthritis (see pp. 64–70) of the spine is another major cause of low back pain. Osteoarthritis pain usually occurs in later life and may involve any part of the spine. Patients often complain of pain, centred about the spine, which is worse in movement and is invariably associated with stiffness and limitation of movement. There is a notable absence of systemic symptoms such as fatigue, malaise or fever, and the pain can usually be relieved by rest.

Usefulness of TENS in Low Back Pain

One of the greatest advances in the management of low back pain has been the introduction of TENS. The use of TENS in the acute phase of the low back strain often provides prompt relief of muscle spasm, rapid control of pain and it greatly accelerates the patients' recovery. The greatest benefits occur when TENS is instituted in the acute phase and used for 1–3 days along with proper instruction in mobility and activity (Ersek 1977; Mannheimer and Lampe 1984).

In recent years a number of studies (Bates and Nathan 1980; Magora et al. 1978; Melzack et al. 1983; Moore and Blacker 1983; Wolf et al. 1981) have reported on the pain-alleviating effect of TENS in chronic low back pain (mainly due to strain). Most studies show that TENS relieves pain effectively ($> 50\%$ pain reduction) in about 50% of patients on a short-term basis (days). The long-term (2-year) results indicate that a limited number of patients (about 20%) continue the use of TENS. Lehmann et al. (1986) reported on 54 patients treated over a 3-week period in a patient rehabilitation programme. The patients were randomly assigned to treatment with electro-acupuncture, low-intensity TENS and placebo TENS. There were no significant differences between treatment groups with respect to their overall rehabilitation. All three treatment groups ranked the contribution of education as being greater than that of electrical stimulation.

Fox and Melzack (1976) compared the effect of acupuncture and TENS in 12 patients suffering chronic low back pain. The authors conclude that both methods appear to be equally effective, but TENS the more practical since it can be administered under supervision by paramedical personnel.

Fried et al. (1984) have reported on the effectiveness of long-term TENS in the treatment of chronic post-traumatic low back pain. Of the 846 patients studied, 45% were free of disability and an additional 36% capable of modified work after TENS treatment. At the 6-month follow-up, most respondents (89%) reported continuing benefit from TENS, a reduction of pain (74%), less need for medication (57%) and improved sleep patterns (59%).

Richardson et al. (1980) reported significant benefit from TENS when used in patients with acute spinal cord injuries. Electrodes were placed on each side of the abdomen on the lower quadrants or paravertebrally at the site of injury, and stimulation was performed constantly for 3 days until bowel movements became apparent or until the patient was virtually pain free. None of the patients developed ileus, gastrointestinal haemorrhage or obstruction. Also, good results have been reported on the use of TENS in chronic spinal cord injuries (Davis and Lentini 1975; Hachen 1978). Furthermore Bajd et al. (1985) have reported that TENS applied proximal to the spastic muscle groups merits consideration in the treatment of spasticity as a result of spinal cord injuries.

## References

Bajd T, Gregoric M, Vodovnik L, Benko H (1985) Electrical stimulation in treating spasticity resulting from spinal cord injury. Arch Phys Med Rehabil 66:515
Bates JAV, Nathan PW (1980) Transcutaneous electrical nerve stimulation for chronic pain. Anaesthesia 35:817
Davis R, Lentini R (1975) Transcutaneous nerve stimulation for treatment of pain in spinal cord injured patients. Surg Neurol 4:100
Ersek RA (1977) Relief of acute musculo-skeletal pain using transcutaneous electrical neuro-stimulation. JACEP 6:300
Fox EJ, Melzack R (1976) Transcutaneous electrical stimulation and acupuncture: comparison of treatment for low back pain. Pain 2:141
Fried T, Johnson R, McCracken W (1984) Transcutaneous electrical nerve stimulation: its role in the control of chronic pain. Arch Phys Med Rehabil 65:228
Hachen HJ (1978) Psychological, neurophysiological and therapeutic aspects of chronic pain-preliminary results with transcutaneous electrical stimulation. Paraplegia 1 25:353
Lehmann TR, Russell DW, Spratt KF, Colby H, Liu YK, Fairchild ML, Christensen S (1986) Efficacy of electroacupuncture and TENS in the rehabilitation of chronic low back pain patients. Pain 2:277
Magora F, Aladjenoff L, Tannenbaum J, Magora A (1978) Treatment of pain by transcutaneous electrical stimulation. Acta anaesthesiol Scand 22:587
Mannheimer JS, Lampe GN (1984) Clinical transcutaneous electrical nerve stimulation. Davis, Philadelphia
Melzack R, Vetere P, Finch L (1983) Transcutaneous electrical nerve stimulation for low back pain: a comparison of TENS and massage for pain and range of motion. Phys Ther 63:489
Moore DE, Blacker HM (1983) How effective is TENS for chronic pain? Am J Nurs 83:1175
Richardson RR, Meyer PR, Cerullo LJ (1980) Transcutaneous electrical neurostimulation in musculoskeletal pain of acute spinal cord injuries. Spine 5:42
Wolf SL, Gersh MR, Rao VR (1981) Examination of electrode placement and stimulating parameters in treating chronic pain with conventional electrical nerve stimulation (TENS). Pain 11:37

## Suggested Reading

Banerjee T (1974) Transcutaneous nerve stimulation for pain after spinal injury. N Engl J Med 29:296
Brill MM, Whiffen JR (1985) Application of 24-hour burst TENS in a back school. Phys Ther 65:1355
Dooley DM, Kasprak M, Stibitz M (1976) Electrical stimulation of the spinal cord in patients with demyelinating and degenerative diseases of the central nervous system. J Fla Med Assoc 63:906
Ersek RA (1976) Low back pain: prompt relief with transcutaneous neurostimulation. Orthop Rev 5:27
Gunn CC, Milbrandt WE (1975) Review of 100 patients with low back sprain treated by surface electrode stimulation of acupuncture points. Am J Acupunct 3:224
Laitinen J (1976) Acupuncture and transcutaneous electric nerve stimulation in the treatment of chronic sacrolumbalgia and ischalgia. Am J Chin Med 4:169

Leyson JFJ, Stefaniwsky L, Martin BF (1979) Effects of transcutaneous nerve stimulation on the vesicourethral function in spinal cord injury patients. J Urol 121:635

Mooney V, Cairns D (1978) Management of the patient with chronic low back pain. Orthop Clin North Am 9:543

Paxton SL (1980) Clinical uses of TENS: a survey of physical therapists. Phys Ther 60:38

Richardson RR, Meyer PR, Raimondi AJ (1979) Transabdominal neurostimulation in acute spinal cord injuries. Spine 4:47

Seres JL, Newman RI (1976) Results of treatment of chronic low back pain at the Portland Pain Center. J Neurosurg 45:32

Walmsley RP, Flexman NE (1979) Transcutaneous nerve stimulation for chronic low back pain: a pilot study. Physiother Can 31:245

Winter A (1976) The use of transcutaneous electrical stimulation (TNS) in the treatment of multiple sclerosis. J Neurosurg Nurs 8:125

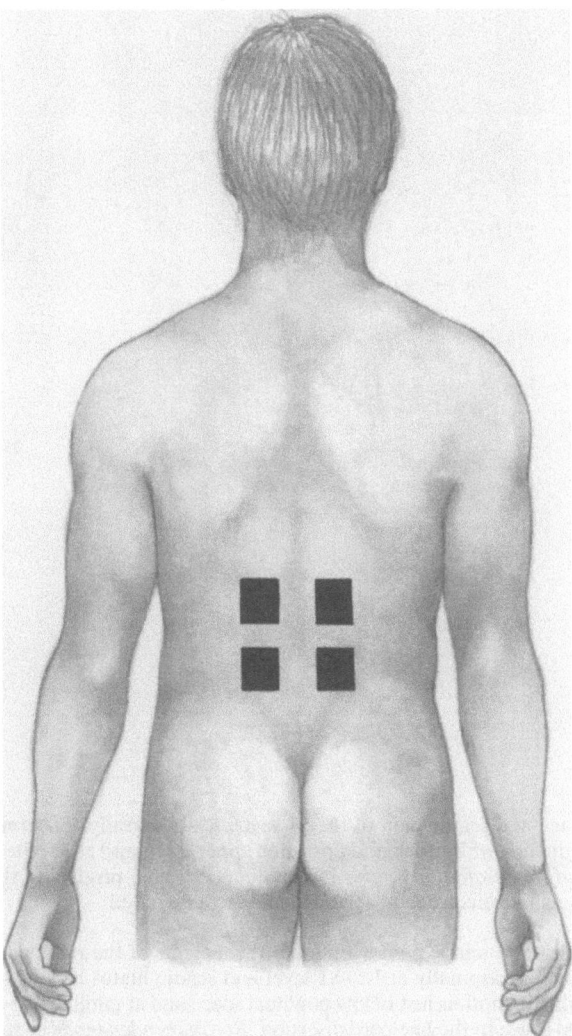

Fig. 3.12. Low back pain after lumbar disc herniation. *Electrode placement sites:* one pair paraspinally and bilaterally at L3 level; another pair paraspinally and bilaterally on left and right at S2 level. *Recommended mode of stimulation:* high frequency, intensity just below pain threshold. *Polarity:* generally of no importance

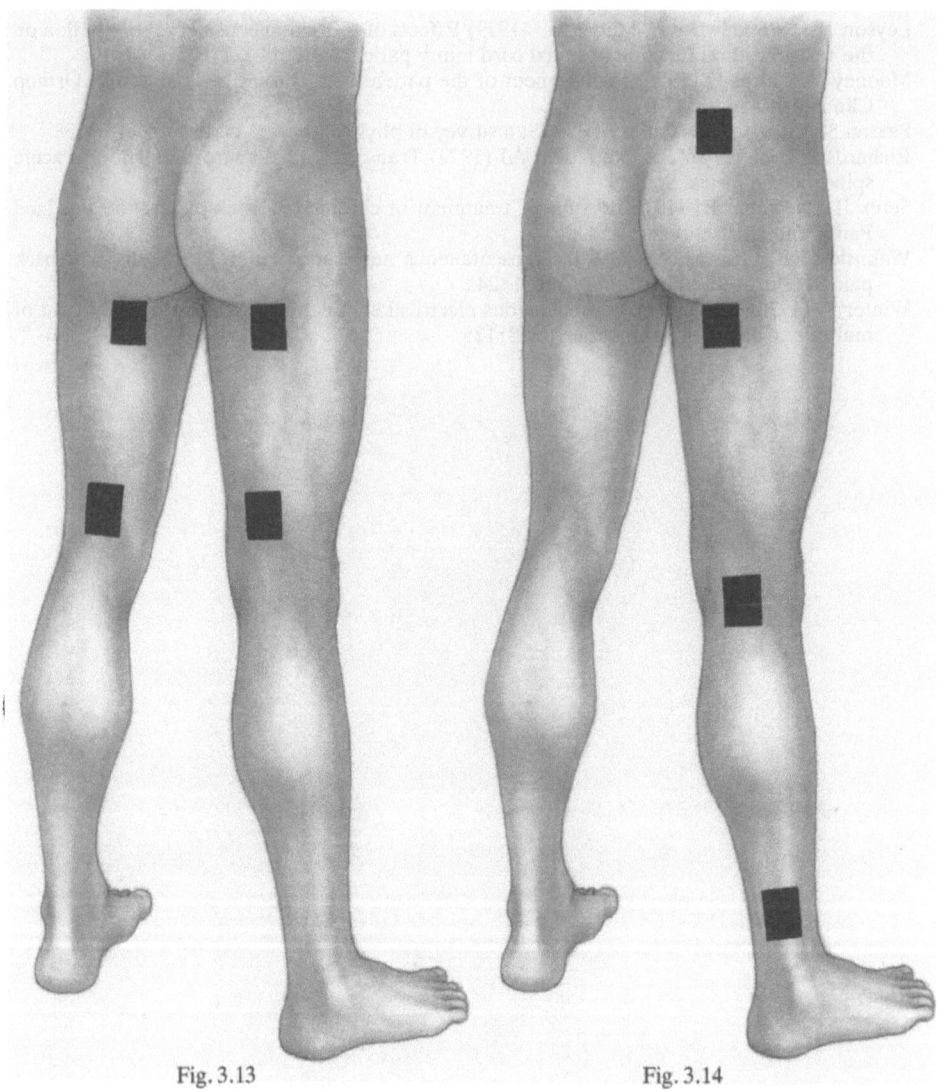

Fig. 3.13.                                    Fig. 3.14.

Fig. 3.13. Low back and sciatic pain of the S1 segments bilaterally. *Electrode placement sites:* sciatic hiatus at junction of buttock and posterior upper thigh and at popliteal space; bilaterally. *Recommended mode of stimulation:* low-frequency trains, producing rhythmical contractions. *Polarity:* negative electrode at sciatic hiatus recommended

Fig. 3.14. Low back and sciatic pain within the S1 segments of the right side. *Electrode placement sites:* one pair paraspinally at L5–S1 level and sciatic hiatus at junction of buttock and posterior upper thigh; another just below popliteal space and at midline two-thirds the distance from the popliteal space to the heelcord insertion. *Recommended mode of stimulation:* low-frequency trains, producing rhythmical contractions. *Polarity:* negative electrodes at sciatic hiatus and just below popliteal space

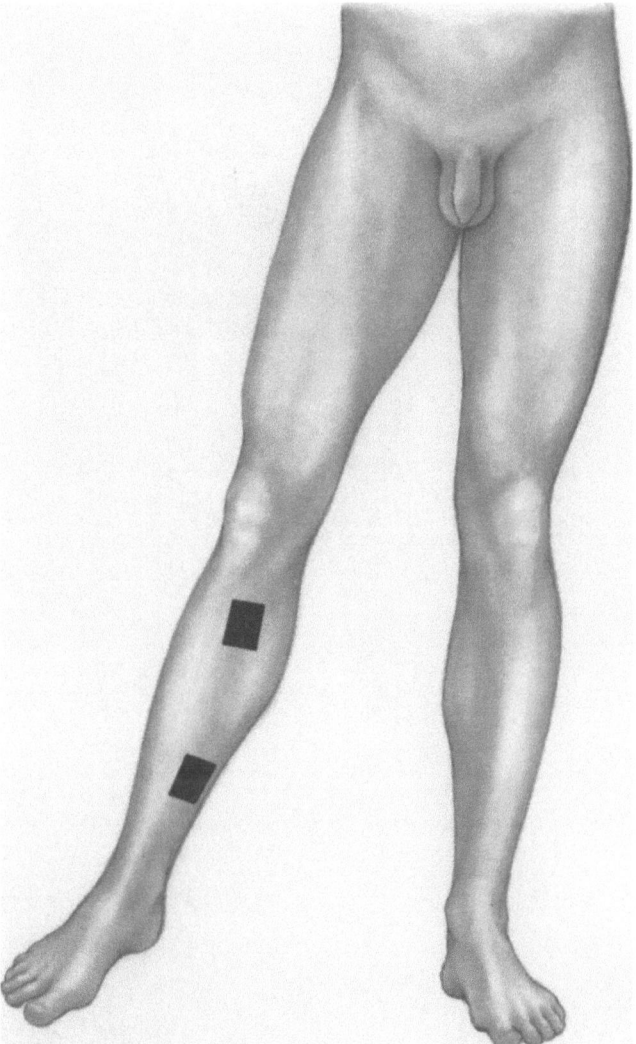

Fig. 3.15. Low back and sciatic pain within the L4 segment on the right side. *Electrode placement sites:* on vastus lateralis and medial head of gastrocnemius. *Recommended mode of stimulation:* high frequency, just below pain threshold. *Polarity:* generally of no importance

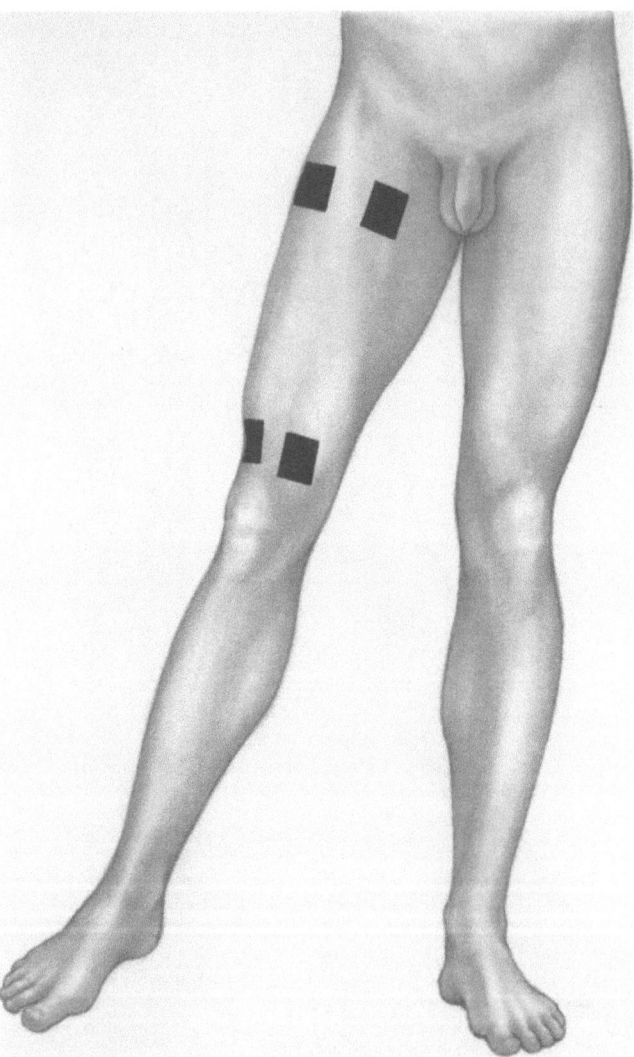

Fig. 3.16. Low back and sciatic pain with impaired sensibility within the L4 segment on the right side. *Electrode placement sites:* one pair on vastus lateralis and adductor magnus; another pair on vastus lateralis and adductor longus. *Recommended mode of stimulation:* low-frequency trains, producing rhythmical contractions. *Polarity:* generally of no importance

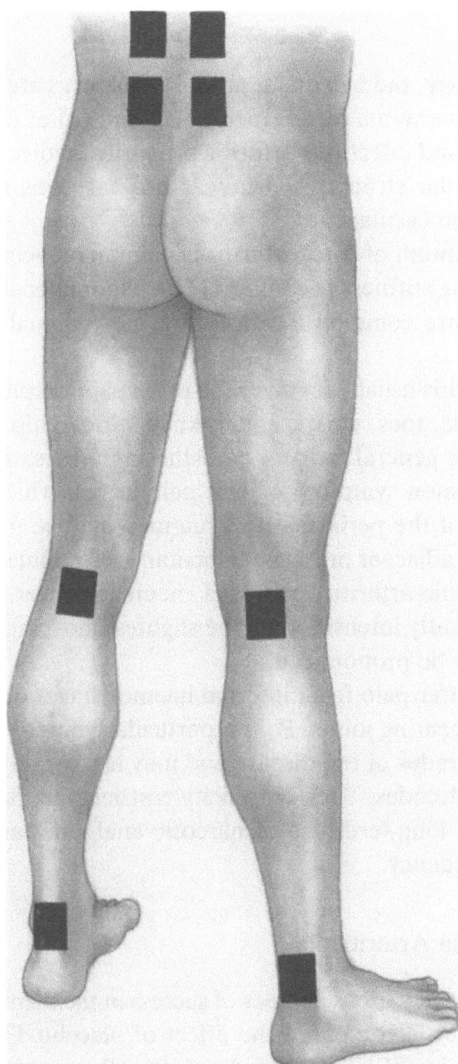

Fig. 3.17. Low back pain with bilateral radiation. *Electrode placement sites:* one pair para-spinally in upper region of low back pain area; another pair just below popliteal crease and at midline two-thirds the distance from the popliteal space to the tendo-achilles insertion. *Recom-mended mode of stimulation:* high-frequency − paraspinal electrodes; low-frequency trains − leg electrodes, intensity set just below pain threshold. *Polarity:* generally of no importance

# Arthritic Pain

Depending on aetiology, the five major groups of arthritis are: (a) infectious; (b) degenerative; (c) post-traumatic; (d) metabolic; and (e) of unknown aetiology. Rheumatoid disease and infectious arthritis primarily involve the synovial membranes and periarticular structures, whereas osteoarthritis and rarer varieties mainly affect bone and cartilage.

The principal symptom of osteoarthritis is pain on movement and is relieved by rest. Early morning stiffness is common, but seldom persists for more than a few minutes. The more common locations are the terminal phalanges, knees, hips and spine.

Rheumatoid arthritis usually involves the proximal interphalangeal and meta-carpophalangeal joints, toes, wrists, ankle, knee, elbow, hip and shoulder. The onset is insidious with general fatigue, paresthesia in the extremities, joint pain and stiffness. A common symptom is joint pain at rest which is aggravated by motion. Thickening of the periarticular structures may be marked and accompanied by atrophy of adjacent muscles. Subcutaneous nodules are often found.

With acute pyogenic arthritis, gout and rheumatic fever, the pain is severe even at rest and is greatly intensified by the slightest movement. Local swelling, redness and heat may be pronounced.

Haemophiliacs suffer pain from internal haemorrhages occurring most commonly in the weight-bearing joints. Pain is particularly intense in those suffering moderate or severe grades of the disease and may last for days or weeks. These episodes recur over decades. Such chronicity restricts the management of pain due to bleeding to a long-term use of narcotic analgesics and the consequent danger of drug dependency.

## Usefulness of TENS in Arthritic Pain

TENS has been used with various degrees of success in the management of arthritic pain. Taylor et al. (1981) compared the effect of placebo TENS and TENS in osteoarthritic knee pain. TENS provided significantly more pain relief than did the placebo in both subjective and medication analyses.

In a study by Lewis et al. (1984) 30 patients with chronic pain due to osteoarthrosis of the knee were enrolled in a randomised double-blind cross-over trial of TENS and placebo TENS. A total of 46% of the patients responded to TENS and 43% to placebo TENS. The length of pain relief due to TENS was significantly longer than that with placebo. At the end of the trial more patients wanted to continue using active TENS in preference to placebo or their original medication. The results of Taylor et al. (1981) and Lewis et al. (1984) are supported by Paxton (1980) and Indeck and Printy (1975). These authors recommend placement of electrodes close to the site of pain (representing sites of innervation of the joint).

In a study by Mannheimer and Carlsson (1979) TENS was used on 20 patients with severe wrist pain due to rheumatoid arthritis. Three different stimulation frequencies were tried: 70-Hz, 3-Hz and 3-Hz trains. The analgesic effect was evaluated by means of a loading time test (pain test) and by the patients' own estimate of pain relief. The results of both evaluations corresponded well. After 70-Hz TENS, 18 patients could double their loading time. The corresponding number for 3-Hz trains TENS was 16 patients and for 3-Hz TENS five patients. The average duration of pain relief after cessation of stimulation was 18 h for 70-Hz TENS and 15 h for 3-Hz trains TENS, while those who responded to 3-Hz TENS experienced pain relief for 4 h on average. In a study by Langley et al. (1984) the analgesic effects of high-frequency TENS, "acupuncture-like" TENS and placebo TENS were evaluated in 33 patients with rheumatoid arthritis of the hands using a randomised, double-blind, non-cross-over design. An oscilloscope was employed to monitor the stimulator output in the TENS treatment groups and to focus attention on the stimulus in the placebo treatment group. The two forms of TENS were applied at the highest intensity that could be tolerated by the patients. Assessments of resting pain, joint tenderness, grip strength and grip pain were made before and after treatment. The pain and joint tenderness measurements showed high-frequency TENS, acupuncture-like TENS and placebo TENS to be equally effective in producing analgesia of similar degree and trend over time. The grip strength measurements showed no significant change.

The use of TENS on haemophiliacs suffering severe joint pain when haemorrhaging was studied by Roche et al. (1985). Thirty-six haemophiliac patients received either active or placebo TENS treatment. The intensity of pain was assessed before and after treatment. After 25 min of active treatment, 26% of the patients reported at least 50% pain relief compared with 9% patients in the placebo group.

## References

Indeck W, Printy A (1975) Skin application of electrical impulses for relief of pain in chronic orthopaedic conditions. Minn Med 58:305

Langley GB, Sheppeard H, Johnsson M, Wigley RD (1984) The analgesic effects of transcutaneous electrical nerve stimulation and placebo in chronic pain patients. A double-blind non-crossover comparison. Rheumatol Int 4:119

Lewis D, Lewis B, Sturrock RD (1984) Transcutaneous electrical nerve stimulation in osteoarthrosis: a therapeutic alternative. Ann Rheum Dis 43:47

Mannheimer C, Carlsson CA (1979) The analgesic effect of transcutaneous electrical nerve stimulation (TNS) in patients with rheumatoid arthritis. A comparative study of different pulse patterns. Pain 6:329

Paxton SL (1980) Clinical use of TENS: a survey of physical therapists. Phys Ther 60:38

Roche PA, Gijsbers K, Belch JJ, Forbes CD (1985) Modification of haemophiliac haemorrhage pain by transcutaneous electrical nerve stimulation. Pain 21:43

Taylor P, Hallett M, Flaherty L (1981) Treatment of osteoarthritis of the knee with transcutaneous electrical stimulation. Pain 11:233

Suggested Reading

Loeser JD, Black RG, Christman A (1975) Relief of pain by transcutaneous stimulation. J
    Neurosurg 42:308
Olm WA, Gold ML, Weil LS (1979) Evaluation of transcutaneous electrical nerve stimulation
    (TENS) in podiatric surgery. J Am Podiatry Assoc 69:537
Shealy CN (1974) Electrical control of the nervous system. Med Prog Technol 2:71

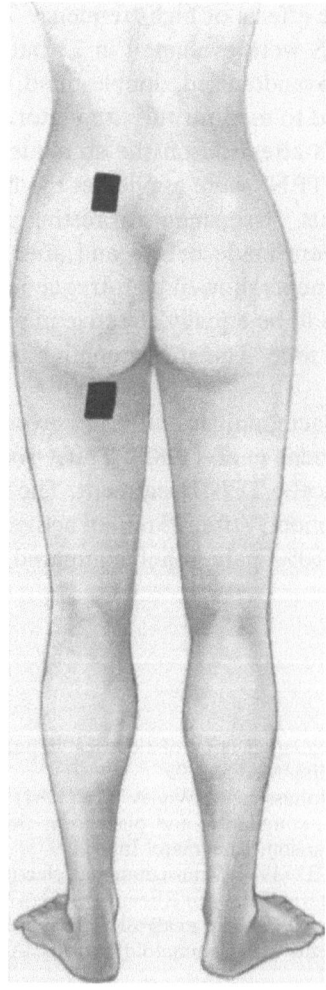

Fig. 3.18. Arthritic pain of sacroiliac joint. *Electrode placement sites:* paraspinally at L5–S1
level and sciatic hiatus at midpoint between ischial tuberosity and greater trochanter. *Recommended mode of stimulation:* high frequency, intensity set just below pain threshold. *Polarity:*
generally of no importance

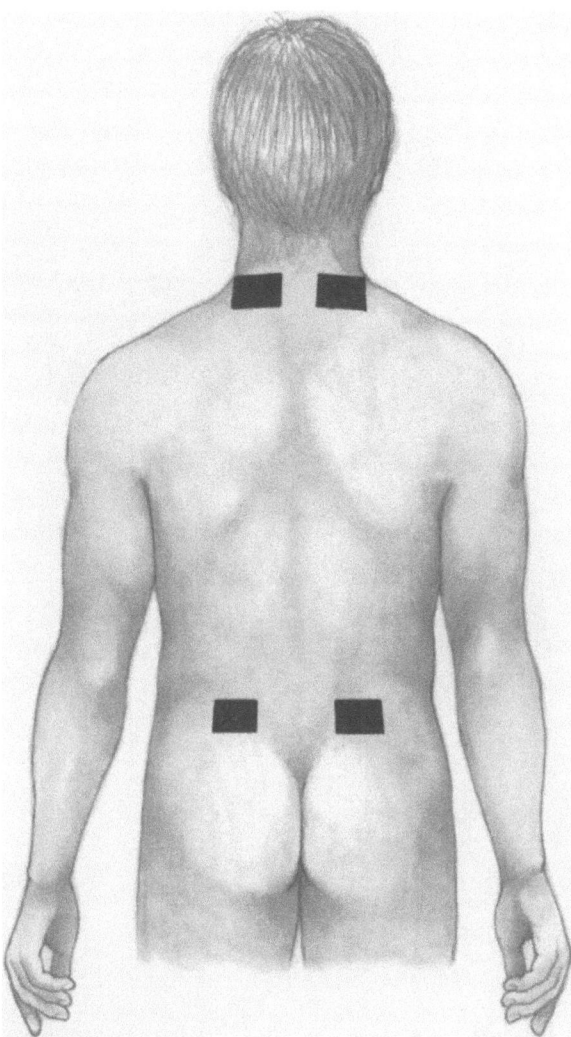

Fig. 3.19. Arthritic pain of cervical and lumbar spine. *Electrode placement sites:* one pair paraspinally at cervicothoracic junction; another pair paraspinally at lumbosacral junction. *Recommended mode of stimulation:* high frequency, intensity set just below pain threshold. *Polarity:* generally of no importance

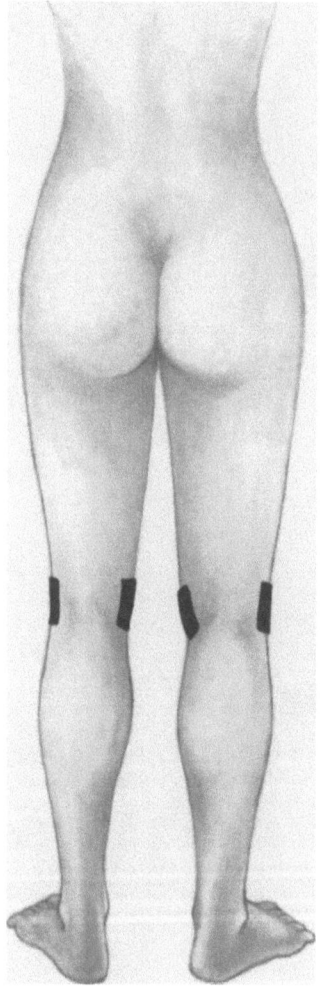

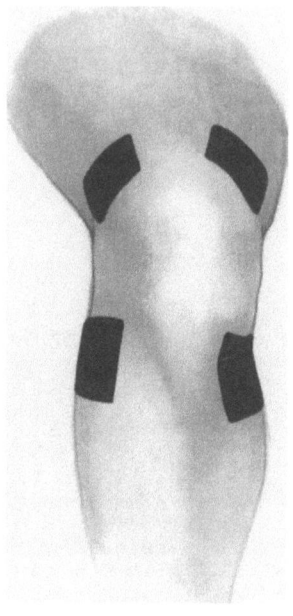

Fig. 3.21

Fig. 3.20

Fig. 3.20. Arthritic knee pain. *Electrode placement sites:* just superior to lateral joint line in depression above femoral condyle and medial joint line between tendons of semitendinosus and semimembranosus. *Recommended mode of stimulation:* high frequency, intensity just below pain threshold. *Polarity:* generally of no importance

Fig. 3.21. Alternative placement of electrodes in knee pain. *Electrode placement sites:* one pair 5 cm above medial aspect of patellar base and anterior-inferior to fibular head; another pair 5 cm above lateral aspect of patellar base and just below medial condyle of tibia. *Recommended mode of stimulation:* high frequency, intensity just below pain threshold. *Polarity:* generally of no importance

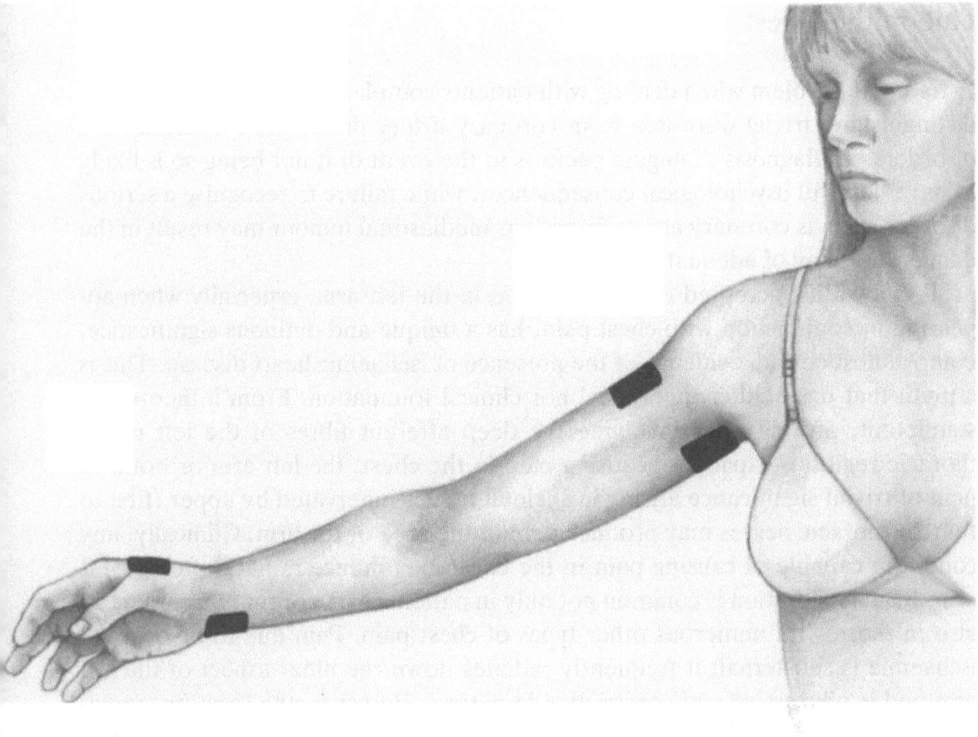

Fig. 3.22. Arthritic pain of wrist. *Electrode placement sites:* dorsal web space and volar surface of wrist. *Recommended mode of stimulation:* high frequency, intensity just below pain threshold. *Polarity:* generally of no importance

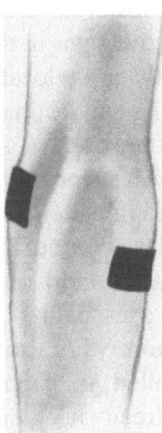

Fig. 3.23. Arthritic pain of elbow. *Electrode placement sites:* in lateral depression at end of elbow crease and just above medial epicondyle and antecubital fossa. *Recommended mode of stimulation:* high frequency, intensity just below pain threshold. *Polarity:* generally of no importance

## Pain in the Chest

A frequent problem when dealing with patients complaining of chest pain lies in distinguishing trivial disorders from coronary artery disease and other serious disorders. A diagnosis of angina pectoris in the event of it not being so is likely to have harmful psychological consequences, while failure to recognise a serious disorder such as coronary artery disease or mediastinal tumour may result in the dangerous delay of adequate treatment.

It is a widely accepted notion that pain in the left arm, especially when appearing in conjunction with chest pain, has a unique and ominous significance, being almost certain evidence of the presence of ischaemic heart disease. This is a myth that has neither theoretical nor clinical foundation. From a theoretical standpoint, any disorder involving the deep afferent fibres of the left upper thoracic region is capable of causing pain in the chest, the left arm or both. A pain of trivial significance arising in skeletal tissues innervated by upper (first to fourth) thoracic nerves may produce pain in the area of the arm. Clinically, any condition capable of causing pain in the chest may induce radiation to the left arm. Such localisation is common not only in patients with coronary disease, but also in those with numerous other types of chest pain. Pain due to myocardial ischaemia is substernal; it frequently radiates down the ulnar aspect of the left arm and is oppressive and constricting in nature. However, the location, radiation and quality of pain are of less diagnostic significance than the behaviour of the pain in terms of the conditions which induce and relieve it.

Only the more important or common conditions causing chest pain that can be treated with TENS will be considered here.

The costochondral and chondrosternal articulations are the most common sites of anterior chest pain. Objective signs in the form of swelling (Tietze's syndrome) and redness are rare, but sharply localised tenderness is common. The pain may be "neuritic", i.e. darting and lasting only a few seconds, or it can be a dull ache which continues for hours or days. An associated feeling of tightness due to muscle spasm is frequent. This type of discomfort is also common in persons with arthritis of the spine and in patients with ischaemic heart disease, but in many instances no such disorder is found. It should be emphasised that palpating the chondrosternal and costochondral junctions is an essential part of the examination of every patient with chest pain. A large percentage of patients with costochondral pain, especially those who also have minor and innocent ECG alterations, are erroneously labelled as having coronary disease. The conse-·quences of such a mistake have already been emphasised.

Chest pain secondary to subacromial bursitis and arthritis of the shoulder or thoracic spine can be precipitated by exercise. It may also be brought about by passive movement of the area involved or by coughing. Prolapsed cervical discs could also cause such pain.

Precordial pain with radiation to the left arm may be due to compression of portions of the brachial plexus by a cervical rib or by spasm and shortening of the scalenus anticus muscle secondary to high fixation of the ribs and sternum.

Skeletal pains in the chest wall or shoulder girdles or arms are recognised fairly easily. Localised tenderness of the affected area is usually present, and the pain is sometimes clearly related to movements involving the painful locus. Deep breathing, turning or twisting of the chest and movements of the shoulder girdle and arm will elicit and duplicate the pain of which the patient complains. The pain may be very brief, lasting only a few seconds, or dull and aching, continuing for hours. Skeletal pains often have a sharp or piercing quality. There is a feeling of tightness which is probably due to spasm of intercostal or pectoral muscles. This may produce the "morning stiffness" seen in so many skeletal disorders. Characteristically such discomfort is abolished by infiltration of the painful areas with local anaesthetics. When chest wall pain is of recent origin and follows trauma, strain, or some unusual activity involving the pectoral muscles, it presents no problem in diagnosis. However, long-standing skeletal pain is frequent in persons who also have angina pectoris. Thus every middle-aged or elderly patient who has long-standing anterior chest wall pain merits careful investigation for the presence of ischaemic heart disease.

Angina pectoris is a pain syndrome resulting from transient myocardial ischaemia. Approximately 80% of all such patients are male. Typically the patient is in his fifties and has substernal pain or discomfort. The pain can vary in intensity and is commonly brought on by exertion or stress. Radiation of the pain to other areas of the trunk, such as shoulder, abdomen, neck or upper arm is possible, and sometimes pain and cramp-like tightness are the only presenting symptoms.

## Usefulness of TENS in Chest Pain

Lundeberg and collaborators (1988, in press) have studied the effect of high-frequency TENS in 40 patients; ten patients with dull ache of the costochondral articulation, 18 with skeletal pain of the chest wall and 12 with strain of the pectoral muscle. Of the 40, 22 patients reported significant alleviation of pain ($> 50\%$ pain reduction) and, of these, 11 reported complete relief of pain.

In a short-term study by Mannheimer et al. (1986) the effect of high-frequency TENS was observed in ten male patients with angina pectoris. The patients had previously been stabilised on long-term maximal oral treatment by nitroglycerine. The TENS treatment was applied in the painful area during an attack, and the effects were measured by means of repeated bicycle ergometer tests. The TENS treatment resulted in an increased working capacity (16%–85%), normalisation of ECG (decreased ST segment depression) and reduced recovery time. No adverse effects were observed. In a long-term study by Mannheimer et al. (1985) patients used the stimulation treatment three times daily for

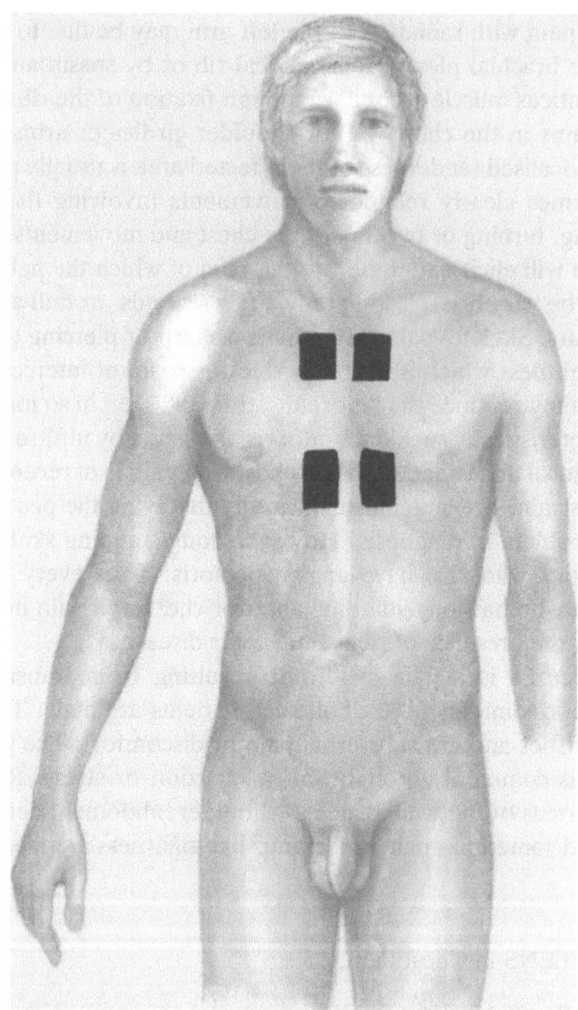

Fig. 3.24. Chondrosternal articulation pain. *Electrode placement sites:* right and left side of the pain area; superior and inferior to the pain area. *Recommended mode of stimulation:* high frequency or low-frequency trains, intensity just below pain threshold. *Polarity:* generally of no importance

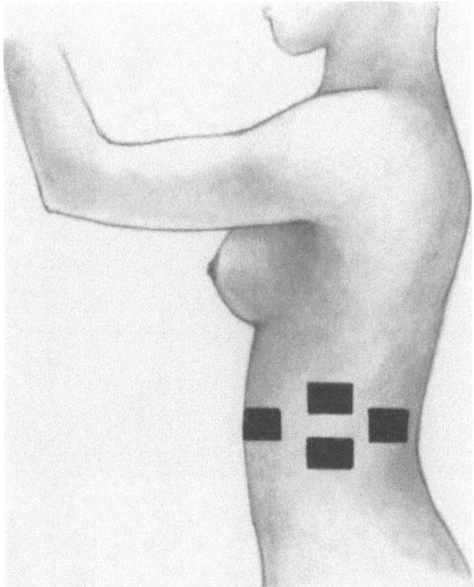

Fig. 3.25. Intercostal neuralgia. *Electrode placement sites:* one pair paraspinal to T6–T10 and at anterior extent of pain; another pair inferior and superior to pain. *Recommended mode of stimulation:* high frequency or low-frequency trains, intensity just below pain threshold. *Polarity:* generally of no importance

1 h at a time and also for 1–10 min during an angina attack. Patients showed beneficial effects in terms of pain reduction, reduced frequency of anginal attacks, increased physical activity and increased working capacity during bicycle ergometer tests.

## References

Mannheimer C, Carlsson CA, Vedin A, Wilhelmsson C (1985) Transcutaneous electrical nerve stimulation (TENS) in angina pectoris. Int J Cardiol 7:91
Mannheimer C, Carlsson CA, Vedin A, Wilhelmsson C (1986) Transcutaneous electrical nerve stimulation (TENS) in angina pectoris. Pain 26:291

## Suggested Reading

Ke-hou D, Xi-hai Y, Ji-min X, Lan-ying S, Wei-bin Z, Fu-pei C (1987) Transcutaneous electrical nerve stimulation (TENS) in 65 severe cases of angina pectoris. Pain [Suppl] 4:371
Myers RMA, Wolf CJ, Mitchell D (1977) Management of acute traumatic pain by peripheral transcutaneous electrical stimulation. S Afr Med J 52:309
Richardson RR, Meyer PR, Raimondi AJ (1979) Transabdominal neurostimulation in acute spinal cord injuries. Spine 4:47
Richardson RR, Meyer PR, Cerullo LJ (1980) Transcutaneous electrical neurostimulation in musculoskeletal pain of acute spinal cord injuries. Spine 5:42
Sovijarvi ARA, Poppius H (1977) Acute bronchodilating effect of TENS in asthma: a peripheral reflex or psychogenic response. Scand J Resp Dis 58:164

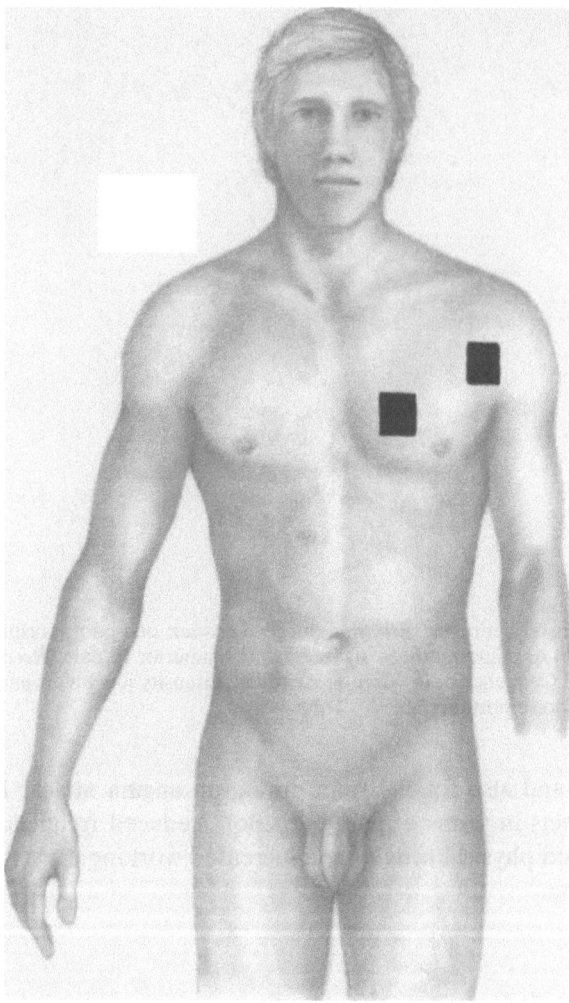

Fig. 3.26. Angina pectoris. *Electrode placement sites:* right and left side of the pain; superior and inferior to pain. *Recommended mode of stimulation:* high frequency, intensity just below pain threshold. *Polarity:* generally of no importance

# Fracture Pain

Fractures are usually associated with point tenderness and oedema at the fracture site, but sometimes pain is referred either proximally or distally. Fracture pain is usually referred in a sclerotomal manner; for instance femoral shaft fracture may refer pain to the hip and knee.

## Usefulness of TENS in Fracture Pain

Sloan et al. (1986) have used TENS to treat the acute pain of rib fractures. The study showed that TENS was as effective as analgesic combinations. Mannheimer and Lampe (1984) have suggested that TENS may be used for the alleviation of fracture pain and in patients who develop reflex sympathetic dystrophy. These patients often need to use TENS on a daily basis. They have also recommended that TENS may have a beneficial effect in fracture healing. They suggest that the electrode placement be arranged so that current flow is across the fracture site.

## References

Mannheimer JS, Lampe GN (1984) Clinical transcutaneous electrical nerve stimulation. Davis, Philadelphia
Sloan JP, Muwanga CL, Waters EA, Dove AF, Dave SH (1986) Multiple rib fractures: transcutaneous nerve stimulation versus conventional analgesia. J Trauma 26:1120–1122

## Suggested Reading

Bassett CAL, Mitchell SN, Gaston SR (1981) Treatment of ununited tibial diaphyseal fractures with pulsing electromagnetic fields. J Bone Joint Surg [Am] 63:511
Batten GB, Lichtman DM (1982) Electricity and bone healing: historical development and review of the literature. Ortho Survey 5:262
Sharrard WJW et al (1982) The treatment of fibrous non-union of fractures by pulsing electromagnetic stimulation. J Bone Joint Surg [Br] 64:189

# Deafferentation Pain

Nerve damage leading to a permanent loss of peripheral sensory nerves produces pain syndromes which are usually categorised as deafferentation pain. These syndromes arise from injuries, any disease associated with nerve degeneration or by surgical interventions resulting in nerve damage. They are classified as neuralgic pain syndromes and include stump and phantom limb pain (see pp. 80–90 for usefulness of TENS), causalgia (post-traumatic), post-herpetic pain and trigeminal neuralgia (see pp. 82–85 for usefulness of TENS). The pain may be due to different causes, but injury to peripheral nerves and nerve degeneration is implicated in all of them. In stump limb pain the formation of a neuroma plays an important role in the development of the pain syndrome. In causalgia the pain is clearly related to nerve injury involving the sympathetic system. In post-herpetic pain there is a selective degeneration of the large myelinated fibres. In trigeminal neuralgia the nerve damage may be less easily identified, but there is often demyelination of the large diameter fibres.

To understand deafferentation pain one must take into account its production by both peripheral and central nervous mechanisms. Ongoing activity in the small fibres of the injured or transected nerve may be one factor. Another may be increased excitability in central afferent pain pathways created by the ongoing or abnormal input.

## Usefulness of TENS in Deafferentation Pain

It has been reported by Parry (1981) that 65% of patients with post-traumatic peripheral nerve pain obtain significant relief with high-frequency TENS. TENS may also increase the ability of the patient to recognise by touch objects and texture differences. The best results were obtained when the electrodes were applied proximal to the level of the lesion.

Eriksson et al. (1979) reported that 34% of patients suffering from neuralgic pain continued the TENS treatment (high-frequency or low-frequency trains) for a period of more than 24 months. Their results parallel those of Bohm (1978) who reported that patients with peripheral nerve injury of the trunk would not be likely responders to TENS while patients with facial neuralgia generally had a better outcome.

Results using TENS for post-herpetic neuralgia are not encouraging. Bates and Nathan (1980) reported only 15% satisfactory alleviation of pain after 2 years whereas Sindou and Keravel (1980) reported 25% satisfactory effect after 1 year's use of TENS. Poor results have also been reported by Bianchetti (1986) and are possibly due to the loss of the afferent pathway normally activated by TENS. However, Eriksson et al. (1979), using both high- and low-frequency train TENS have reported more satisfactory results.

It has been reported by several authors (Bohm 1978; Cauthen and Renner 1975; Meyer and Fields 1972; Stilz et al. 1977) that TENS can be tried in patients suffering from reflex sympathetic dystrophy or causalgia. In a long-term study of TENS in causalgia by Parry (1981) 38 out of 70 patients reported that high-frequency TENS for several hours per day produced satisfactory pain relief. Electrodes were placed ipsilateral and proximal to the lesion. Tender points within the painful area as well as paraspinal sites were stimulated.

# References

Bates JAV, Nathan PW (1980) Transcutaneous electrical nerve stimulation for chronic pain. Anaesthesia 35:817

Bianchetti L (1986) La terapia farmacologica della cosiddetta neuralgia post-herpetica unica valida alternativa. Esperienza clinica di 43 casi trattati. Minerva Med 77:47

Bohm E (1978) Transcutaneous electrical nerve stimulation in the chronic pain after peripheral nerve injury. Acta Neurochir (Wien) 40:277

Cauthen JC, Renner EJ (1975) Transcutaneous and peripheral nerve stimulation for chronic pain states. Surg Neurol 4:102

Eriksson MBE, Sjölund BH, Neilzen S (1979) Long term results of peripheral conditioning stimulation as analgesic measure in chronic pain. Pain 6:335

Meyer GA, Fields HC (1972) Causalgia treated by selective large fiber stimulation of peripheral nerve. Brain 95:163

Parry CBW (1981) Rehabilitation of the hand, 4th edn. Butterworths, London, p 129

Sindou M, Keravel Y (1980) Analgésie par la méthode d'électrostimulation transcutaneé. Résultats dans la douleur d'origine neurologique. A propos de 180 cas. Neurochirurgie 26:153

Stilz RJ, Carron H, Sanders DB (1977) Case history number 96: reflex sympathetic dystrophy in a 6 year old: successful treatment by transcutaneous nerve stimulation. Anesth Analg 56:438

# Selected Reading

Parry CBW (1980) Pain in avulsion lesion of the brachial plexus. Pain 9:41

Richlin DM, Carron H, Rowlingson JC (1978) Reflex sympathetic dystrophy: successful treatment by TENS. J Pediatr 93:84

Sternschein JM et al (1975) Causalgia. Arch Phys Med Rehabil 56:58

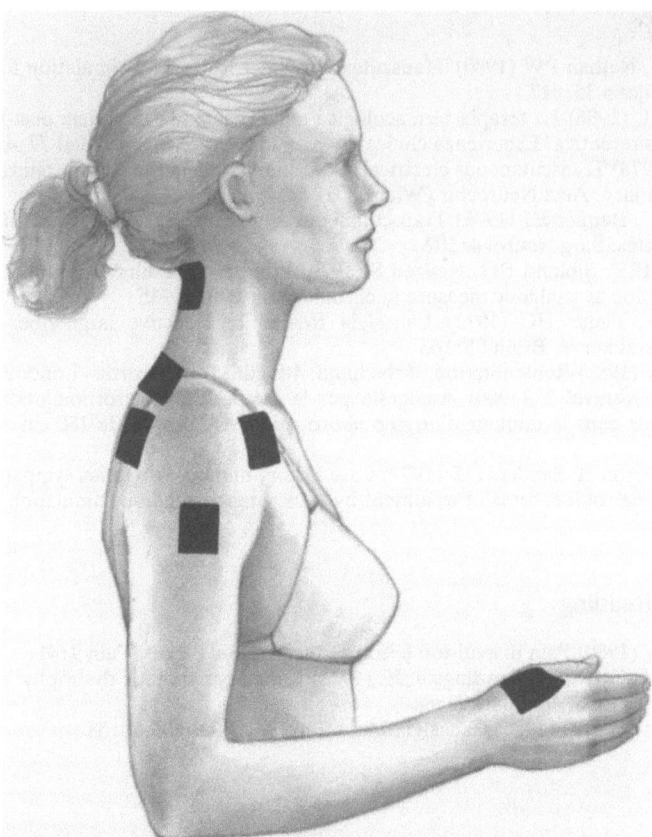

Fig. 3.27. Reflex sympathetic dystrophy. *Electrode placement sites:* one pair lateral to cervical spine, suboccipital to C6 and supraspinous fossa; another pair in depression posterior to acromion and in depression anterior to acromion; insertion of deltoid and dorsal web space. *Recommended mode of stimulation:* high frequency, intensity just below pain threshold. *Polarity:* generally of no importance

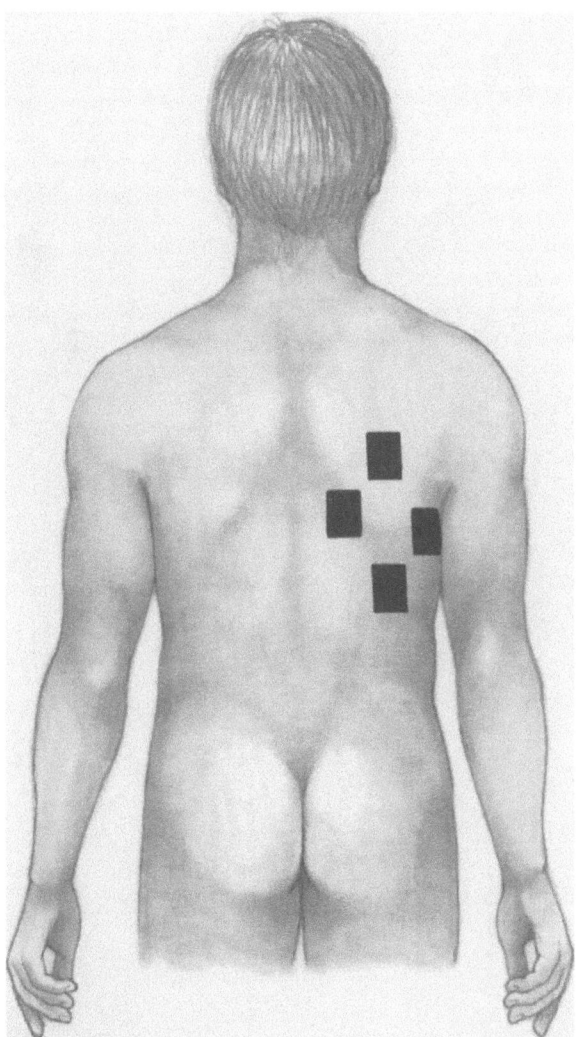

Fig. 3.28. Post-herpetic neuralgia at T6–7 segmental level on the right side; skin sensitivity not reduced. *Electrode placement sites:* in the dermatome just above or above or below the affected segments. *Recommended mode of stimulation:* high frequency, intensity just below pain threshold. *Polarity:* generally of no importance

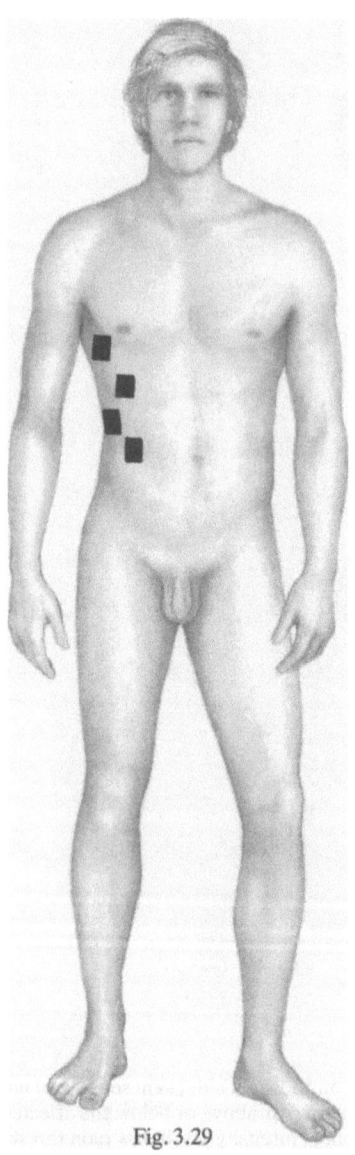

Fig. 3.29

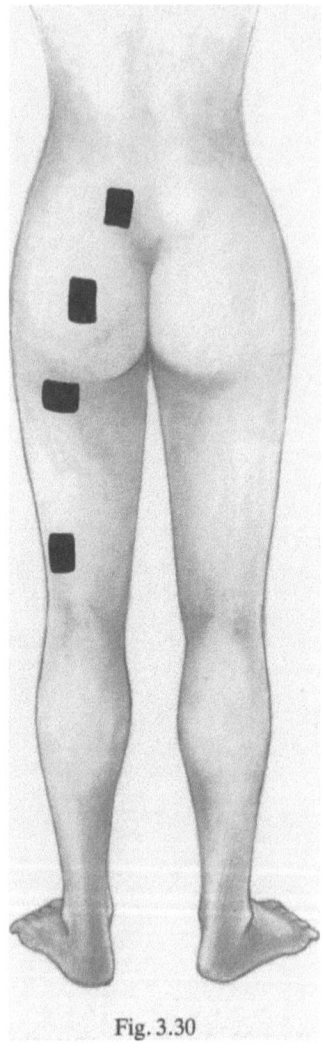

Fig. 3.30

Fig. 3.29. Post-herpetic neuralgia at T6–7 segmental level on the right side (impaired skin sensitivity). *Electrode placement sites:* above and below the affected dermatomes, stimulus intensity should be set to elicit forceful muscle contractions in T6–7 intercostal muscles. *Recommended mode of stimulation:* low frequency, producing rhythmical contractions. *Polarity:* generally of no importance

Fig. 3.30. Post-herpetic neuralgia of sciatic nerve. *Electrode placement sites:* one pair paravertebrally at L5–S1 level and on tender buttock motor point; another pair at midpoint between ischial tuberosity and greater trochanter, and just superior to popliteal crease. *Recommended mode of stimulation:* high frequency, intensity just below pain threshold. *Polarity:* generally of no importance

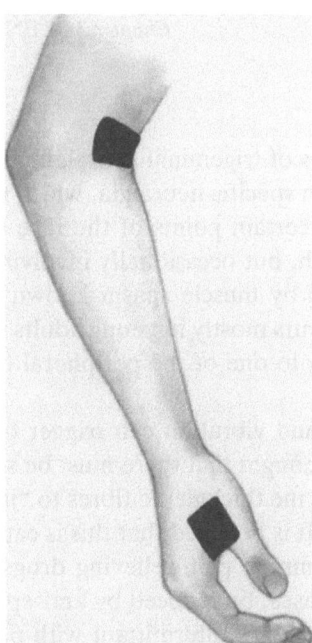

Fig. 3.31. Deafferentation pain of right radial nerve. *Electrode placement sites:* in depression at lateral end of elbow and dorsal web space. *Recommended mode of stimulation:* high frequency or low-frequency trains, intensity just below pain threshold or rhythmical contractions. *Polarity:* generally of no importance

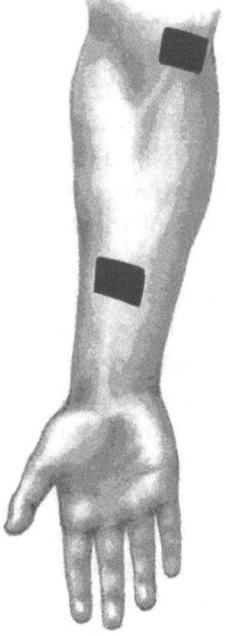

Fig. 3.32 Deafferentation pain of right medial nerve. *Electrode placement sites:* in antecubital fossa lateral to biceps tendon and at volar aspect of wrist. *Recommended mode of stimulation:* high frequency or low-frequency trains, intensity just below pain threshold. *Polarity:* generally of no importance

## Trigeminal Neuralgia

There are two distinct types of trigeminal neuralgia, or facial pain syndromes —
specific and non-specific. In specific neuralgia, which generally presents in older
age, the lightest touch on certain points of the face (usually localised in areas
around the nose and mouth, but occasionally involving the scalp or teeth) trig-
gers intense pain followed by muscle spasm known as tic douloureux). Non-
specific or atypical pain occurs mostly in young adults with an antecedent history
of facial trauma and injury to one of the peripheral branches of the trigeminal
nerve.

Since pressure, touch and vibration can trigger off pain attacks in specific
trigeminal neuralgia, it is thought that there must be some sort of "short circuit"
which causes the activity in the thick nerve fibres to "jump over" to the thin pain
nerves (efaptic overflow). It is believed that this is caused by demyelinisation of
the thick nerve fibres. Common pain-relieving drugs have proved ineffective.
The attacks can, in some cases, be reduced by anti-epileptics.

Attacks of tic douloureux are intermittant with pain-free intervals between
clusters of attacks. Although spontaneous remissions occur and can last for
years, they are not predictable, and episodes can become more frequent and
more intense as years go by. Pain is unilateral with minimal or no sensory loss in
the trigeminal distribution, and the trigger points are ipsilateral to the pain. The
onset and termination are abrupt, but the pain is so severe that it can lead to
total disruption of daily routines of facial and oral hygiene. Those patients with
pain triggered by chewing or swallowing may be unable to ingest sufficient food
to meet their caloric needs. Depression can lead to suicide in the poorly managed patient. Alleviation of symptoms almost always results in prompt restoration of normal mood and behaviour. Retrogasserian injection of glycerol
(Håkansson 1981) may produce complete relief of symptoms and the restoration
of a healthy life pattern.

Patients with non-specific or atypical trigeminal neuralgia often have significant behavioural and psychological dysfunctions that are often shown to have
been present prior to the origin of the facial pain. The pain is often bilateral and
continuous, usually with sensory loss which is not progressive. The severity of
the pain is not as great as in tic douloureux and seldom interrupts normal daily
activities. The symptoms of atypical neuralgia are amazingly constant over time,
medical therapy is rarely effective, and denervating operations usually make the
patient's pain more severe. However, the nature of the pain, coupled with per-
sonality traits, frequently leads to iatrogenic drug abuse. Over the years the patient seems to manifest a less florid pain behaviour, but somatic preoccupation,
passive lifestyle and depression remain. Patients with atypical trigeminal neuralgia
are often a source of great frustration to pain clinics, neurologists and neuro-
surgeons.

## Usefulness of TENS in Trigeminal Neuralgia

Observations of Eriksson et al. (1984) indicate that TENS (high or low-frequency trains) may be a relevant alternative to surgical procedures in specific trigeminal neuralgia (tic douloureux), especially in the elderly where surgical risks are more significant. The results of Eriksson et al. (1984) are clearly superior to those of Thoden and Krainick (1974) and Gregg (1978) who reported about 20% satisfactory pain alleviation at the 6-month follow-up. This may be due to the fact that the latter tried only high-frequency TENS.

Eriksson et al. (1984) and Ihalainen and Perkki (1978) have shown that TENS may be used with satisfactory results in non-specific trigeminal neuralgia (atypical facial pain). This is interesting to note as surgical results are not encouraging in this group of patients.

## References

Eriksson M, Sjölund B, Sundbärg G (1984) Pain relief from peripheral conditioning stimulation in patients with intractable facial pain. J Neurosurg 61:149

Gregg JM (1978) Post-traumatic trigeminal neuralgia: response to physiologic, surgical and pharmacologic therapies. Int Dent J 28:43

Håkansson S (1981) Trigeminal neuralgia treated by the injection of glycerol into the trigeminal cistern. Neurosurgery 9:638

Ihalainen U, Perkki K (1978) The effect of transcutaneous nerve stimulation (TNS) on chronic facial pain. Proc Finn Dent Soc 74:86

Thoden V, Krainick JU (1974) Ambulante Schmerzbehandlung durch transkutane Nervenstimulation. Dtsch Med Wochenschr 99:1692

## Suggested Reading

Cauthen JC, Renner EJ (1975) Transcutaneous and peripheral nerve stimulation for chronic pain states. Surg Neurol 4:102

Ignelzi RJ, Sternbach RA, Callaghan M (1979) Somatosensory changes during transcutaneous electrical analgesia. In: Bonica JJ, Albe-Fessard D (eds) Advances in pain research and therapy, vol 1. Raven, New York, p 509

Kirsch WM, Lewis JA, Simon RH (1975) Experiences with electrical stimulation devices for the control of chronic pain. Med Instrum 9:217

Loeser JD, Black RG, Christman A (1975) Relief on pain by transcutaneous stimulation. J Neurosurg 42:308

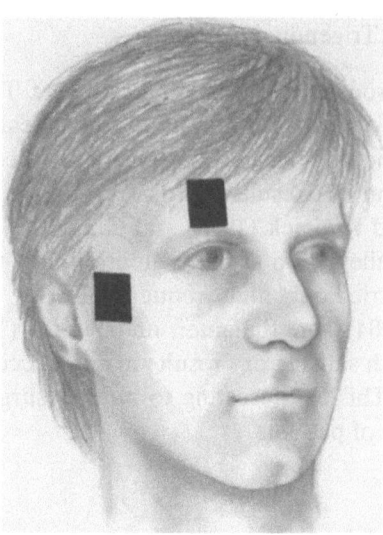

Fig. 3.33. Non-specific trigeminal neuralgia of the first trigeminal nerve branch. *Electrode placement sites:* one electrode supraorbitally and one in front of the ear over the tempero-mandibular joint. *Recommended mode of stimulation:* high frequency if the skin sensitivity is normal; low-frequency trains if sensitivity is reduced, intensity just below pain threshold. *Polarity:* when using high frequency, the negative electrode should be positioned in front of the external ear and the positive electrode on the affected first trigeminal branch. When using low-frequency trains, the reversed polarity is recommended

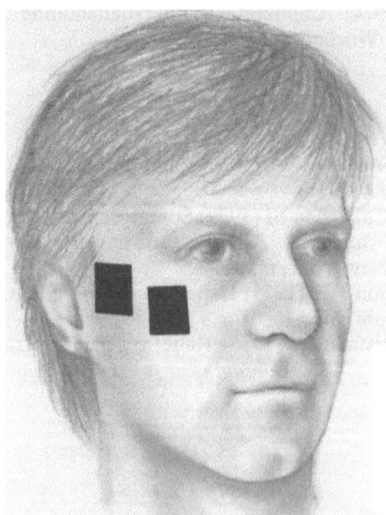

Fig. 3.34. Non-specific trigeminal neuralgia of the second trigeminal nerve branch. *Electrode placement sites:* one electrode in front of the ear over the temperomandibular joint and one electrode infraorbitally. *Recommended mode of stimulation:* high frequency if the skin sensitivity is normal; low-frequency trains if sensitivity is reduced. Intensity just below pain threshold. *Polarity:* When using high frequency, the negative electrode should be positioned in front of the external ear and the positive electrode on the affected first trigeminal branch. When using low-frequency trains, the reversed polarity is recommended

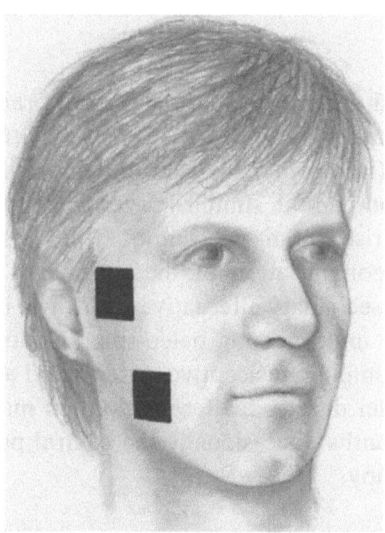

Fig. 3.35. Non-specific trigeminal neuralgia of the third trigeminal nerve branch. *Electrode placement sites:* one electrode in front of the ear over the temperomandibular joint and one electrode on masseter muscle. *Recommended mode of stimulation:* high frequency if the skin sensitivity is normal; low-frequency trains if sensitivity is reduced, intensity just below pain threshold. *Polarity:* when using high frequency, the negative electrode should be positioned in front of the external ear and the positive electrode on the affected first trigeminal branch. When using low-frequency trains, the reversed polarity is recommended

# Central Pain

Central pain occurs with injuries to the spinal cord, brain stem or the thalamus involving the sensory pathways. Pain can be caused by trauma or haemorrhage, or may follow surgery (iatrogenic). Attacks of pain occur spontaneously and as an overreaction to non-painful stimuli. Several mechanisms probably work simultaneously to give rise to the spectrum of symptoms of central pain. These include pathological reorganisation of the sensibility of the spared sensory fibres, development of secondary alternative pathways, irritation of central grey masses or non-specific multisynaptic paleo-spinothalamic systems, loss of inhibitory mechanisms damping nociceptive systems and abnormal firing patterns of central sensory nuclei due to deafferentation. In many cases the condition subsides within 1–2 months. Occasionally the central pain remains and is then highly resistant to therapy.

## Usefulness of TENS in Central Pain

Eriksson et al. (1979) have reported that nine of 18 patients suffering central pain treated with low- or high-frequency TENS experienced useful analgesia at the 12-month follow-up. These results are clearly superior to those reported by Bates and Nathan (1980; 16%) and Sindou and Keravel (1980; 0%–11%). The latter tried only high-frequency TENS. Patients suffering from diffuse body pain as a result of lesions in the thalamus or thalamic pain syndromes do not respond well to TENS (Long 1976).

## References

Bates JAV, Nathan PW (1980) Transcutaneous electrical nerve stimulation for chronic pain. Anaesthesia 35:817
Eriksson MBE, Sjölund BH, Neilzen S (1979) Long term results of peripheral conditioning stimulation as analgesic measure in chronic pain. Pain 6:335
Long DM (1976) Cutaneous afferent stimulation for the relief of pain. Prog Neurol Surg 7:35
Sindou M, Keravel Y (1980) Analgésie par le méthode d'électrostimulation transcutanée. Résultats dans les douleurs d'origine neurologique. A propos de 180 cas. Neurochirurgie 26:153

## Suggested Reading

Kirsch WM, Lewis JA, Simon RH (1975) Experiences with electrical stimulation devices for the control of chronic pain. Med Instrum 9:217
Long DM, Hagfors N (1975) Electrical stimulation of the nervous system: the current status of electrical stimulation of the nervous system for relief of pain. Pain 1:109
Sjölund BH, Eriksson MBE (1980) Stimulation techniques in the management of pain. In: Kosterlitz HW, Terenius LY (eds) Pain and society. Life Sciences Report 17. Weinheim, Deerfield Beach, FL, p 415

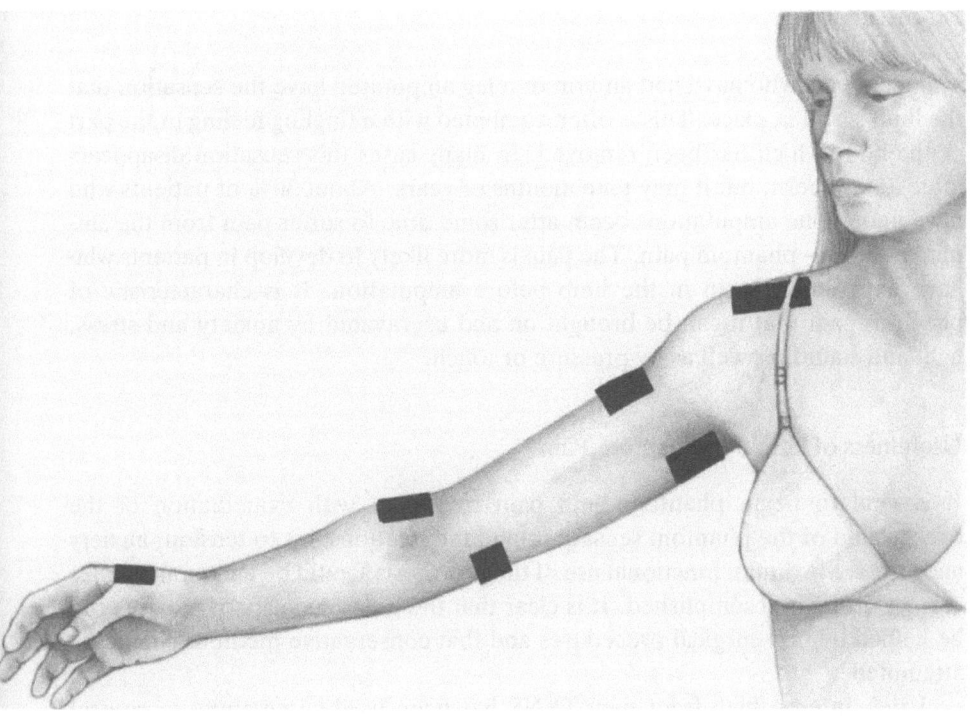

Fig. 3.36. Central pain radiating in the right arm. Electrode placement sites: (a) in depression bordered by the acromion laterally, spine of scapula posteriorly and clavicle anteriorly; (b) insertion of deltoid; (c) lower axilla, medial to brachial artery; (d) just below groove between medial epicondyle and olecranon; (e) 8–10 cm above radial styloid; (f) dorsal web place. The electrodes should be positioned over large nerve bundles in the part of the body where the pain is the most pronounced. At times, stimulation of the contralateral side of the body is effective. Generally multi-channel stimulation is recommended. *Recommended mode of stimulation:* high frequency or low-frequency trains, intensity below pain threshold. *Polarity:* generally of no importance

## Phantom Pain

Many patients who have had an arm or a leg amputated have the sensation that the limb is still in place. This is often combined with a tingling feeling in the part of the body which has been removed. In many cases this sensation disappears after some weeks, but it may take months or years. About 30% of patients who have undergone amputations begin after some time to suffer pain from the amputated limb – phantom pain. The pain is more likely to develop in patients who have experienced pain in the limb before amputation. It is characteristic of phantom pain that it can be brought on and aggravated by anxiety and stress, light and sound, as well as by pressure or touch.

### Usefulness of TENS in Phantom Pain

It is vital to begin phantom limb pain treatment with examination of the background of the phantom sensations and the relationships to tension, anxiety and stress. Maximum functional use of the prosthesis should be encouraged after correct fitting is accomplished. It is clear that the great majority of patients can be helped by non-surgical procedures and that conservative methods should be attempted.

Brief, intense high-frequency TENS has been used successfully to control phantom limb pain (Long 1973). Electrodes were placed on painful trigger points, related peripheral nerves and spinal cord segments innervating the painful area. In some patients, contralateral stimulation was helpful, as were electrodes placed on the skin within the prosthesis (Gyory and Caine 1977; Miles and Lipton 1978). Beneficial effects of TENS in phantom pain have also been reported by Thoden et al. (1979) and Winnem and Amundsen (1982).

Gessler and Struppler (1981) used TENS in ten patients suffering from chronic, cramp-like (flexor muscle) phantom pain. They applied TENS to the nerves innervating the corresponding extensor muscles and reported pain relief in all patients. The patients stated that they felt an opening of the cramp-like flexion. Best results were obtained with 100-Hz TENS and at an intensity of 5–20 mA. Stimulation of the nerves to the flexor muscle increased the phantom pain.

### References

Gessler M, Struppler A (1981) Relief of phantom pain by stimulation of the nerve supplying the corresponding extensor muscles. Pain [Suppl I]:257
Gyory AN, Caine DC (1977) Electric pain control (EPC) of a painful forearm amputation stump. Med J Aust 2:156
Long DM (1973) Electrical stimulation for relief of pain from chronic nerve injury. J Neurosurg 39:718
Miles J, Lipton S (1978) Phantom limb pain treated by electrical stimulation. Pain 5:373

Thoden U, Gruber RP, Krainick J-U, Huber-Muck L (1979) Langzeitergebnisse transkutaner
    Nervenstimulation bei chronisch neurogen Schmerzzuständen. Nervenarzt 50:179
Winnem MF, Amundsen T (1982) Treatment of phantom limb pain with transcutaneous elec-
    trical nerve stimulation. Pain 12:299

## Suggested Reading

Gunn CC (1978) Transcutaneous neural stimulation, acupuncture and the current of injury.
    Am J Acupunct 6:191
Gunn CC (1979) Causalgia and denervation supersensitivity. Am J Acupunct 7:317
Gunn CC (1980) "Prespondylosis" and some pain syndromes following denervation super-
    sensitivity. Spine 5:185
Indeck W, Printy A (1975) Skin application of electrical impulses for relief of pain in chronic
    orthopaedic conditions. Minn Med 58:305
Long DM (1973) Electrical stimulation for relief of pain from chronic nerve injury. J Neuro-
    surg 39:718
Long DM, Hagfors N (1975) Electrical stimulation of the nervous system: The current status
    of electrical stimulation of the nervous system for relief of pain. Pain 1:109

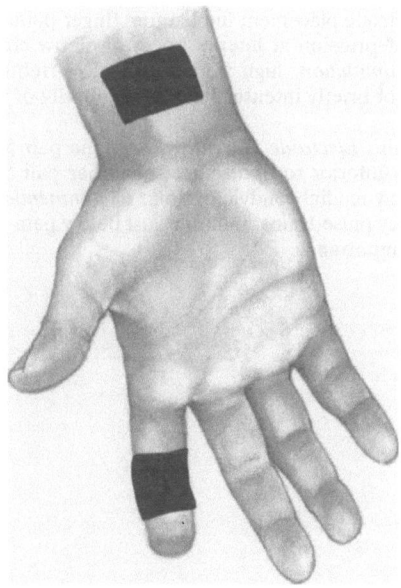

Fig. 3.37. Phantom finger pain of right second finger (traumatic amputation of distal phalanx).
*Electrode placement sites:* volar surface of right wrist and volar surface of right index finger just
proximal to the proximal joint. *Recommended mode of stimulation:* high frequency or low-frequency pulse-trains, intensity just below pain threshold or briefly intense. *Polarity:* generally
of no importance (see also Fig. 3.38)

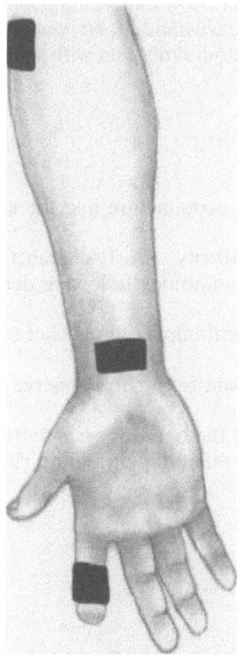
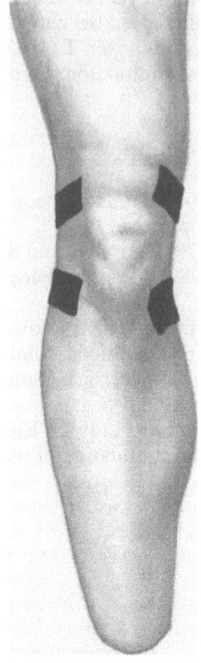

Fig. 3.38                                    Fig. 3.39

Fig. 3.38. Alternative electrode placement in phantom finger pain of right second finger. *Electrode placement sites:* in depression at lateral aspect of elbow crease and dorsal web space. *Recommended mode of stimulation:* high frequency or low-frequency pulse-trains, intensity just below pain threshold or briefly intense. *Polarity:* generally of no importance

Fig. 3.39. Phantom leg pain. *Electrode placement sites:* one pair 5 cm above medial aspect of patellar base and anterior-inferior to fibular head; another pair 5 cm above lateral aspect of patellar base and just below medial condyle of tibia. *Recommended mode of stimulation:* high frequency or low-frequency pulse-trains, intensity just below pain threshold or briefly intense. *Polarity:* generally of no importance

# Vascular Pain

It is not uncommon that patients suffer from pain of vascular origin. The pain may derive from pathological processes within the walls of the arteries or the veins as well as being secondary to some general disorder.

Atherosclerosis of large- and medium-sized arteries is the most common vascular disease in man and leads to symptoms induced by exercise (intermittent claudication), but may also occur at rest (ischaemic rest pain). Pain brought on by exercise and promptly relieved by rest most frequently involves the calf and thigh muscles. Pain at rest is characteristically worse at night and is totally or partially relieved by exercise. Ischaemic rest pain, and the sometimes attendant ulceration and gangrene, is mostly localised to the foot and toes and is usually the result of multiple sites of vascular occlusion.

Another frequent location of vascular pain is in the walls of the veins. The common varieties of inflammation and thrombosis (thrombophlebitis) of the superficial and deep veins following prolonged bed rest, trauma or malignancy may produce pain in the extremities. When superficial veins are involved, the afflicted areas are tender and firm, with associated oedema and erythema of the overlying skin. When the deep veins are involved, generalised aching pain, swelling and/or brawny induration are common.

A general symmetrical disorder of unknown origin is Raynaud's disease. It is benign and usually commences in the late teens or early twenties. Females are the most commonly afflicted, and cold and emotional stimuli are the factors which trigger the response in the digits. The fingers become white, then blue and finally red (the triphasic colour response). Pain and paraesthesias are common during the ischaemic phase. Ulcerations are rarely observed.

Another disorder also carrying Raynaud's name is Raynaud's phenomenon. It is always secondary to some generalised malfunction and is often the first symptom of this condition. The onset is at any period of life and may be unilateral. Excessive use of the hands (e.g. sculling, working with a pneumatic drill) may give rise to Raynaud's phenomenon. When severe it is accompanied by tender, painful, fingertip ulcers. The common disorders associated with this problem are connective tissue disorders such as collagen vascular disease or rheumatoid arthritis, drug intoxications (ergot), thrombo-angitis obliterans, occupational trauma and the thoracic outlet syndrome.

Usefulness of TENS in Vascular Pain

Eriksson and Mannheimer (1980) used TENS in 11 patients who had severe arterial insufficiency of the lower extremities. TENS was performed for 5 min at 80 Hz with an intensity that produced slight vibrations radiating down the calf to the foot. Patients were tested on a treadmill prior to TENS until pain became severe. All patients were able to increase their walking distance after TENS, and seven patients reported that the aching disappeared after TENS.

Roberts (1979) used TENS to manage the pain of thrombophlebitis in the legs of 39 patients. Electrodes were placed over the painful venous segment and its peripheral nerve. Treatments were performed bilaterally if both extremities were involved. Conventional TENS stimulation was performed for 30–60 min, three to four times, over a period of 1–3 days. Good relief was obtained by 32 patients, three obtained fair relief and four had no relief. The patients were cautioned not to stand immediately after pain relief but to resume their normal activities gradually.

Kaada (1982) has reported that low-frequency train TENS can be used with good result in the treatment of patients suffering from Raynaud's phenomenon. TENS applied on an acupuncture point located at the first dorsal web space resulted in a significant peripheral vasodilation with a concommittant skin temperature increase of 7°–10°C in the cold extremity. The increase in skin temperature lasted for at least 4–8 h and was accompanied by the relief of ischaemic pain. It has recently been discovered by Kjartansson and Lundeberg (1987, unpublished results) and Lundeberg (1987, unpublished results) that TENS may increase the peripheral circulation in surgical flaps and leg ulcers as will be described later (pp. 124, 125).

### References

Eriksson H, Mannheimer C (1980) The effect of transcutaneous electric nerve stimulation on ischemic pain in the lower extremities. Gerontal 10:33
Kaada B (1982) Vasodilation induced by transcutaneous nerve stimulation in peripheral ischemia (Raynaud's phenomenon and diabetic polyneuropathy) Eur Heart J 3:303
Roberts HJ (1979) TENS in the symptomatic management of thrombophlebitis. Angiology 30:249

### Suggested Reading

Abram SE (1976) Increased sympathetic tone associated with transcutaneous electrical stimulation. Anesthesiology 45:575
Dooley DM, Kasprak M (1976) Modification of blood flow to the extremities by electrical stimulation of the nervous system. South Med J 69:1309
Schuster GD (1980) The use of TENS for peripheral neurovascular diseases. J Neurol Orthop Surg 1:219

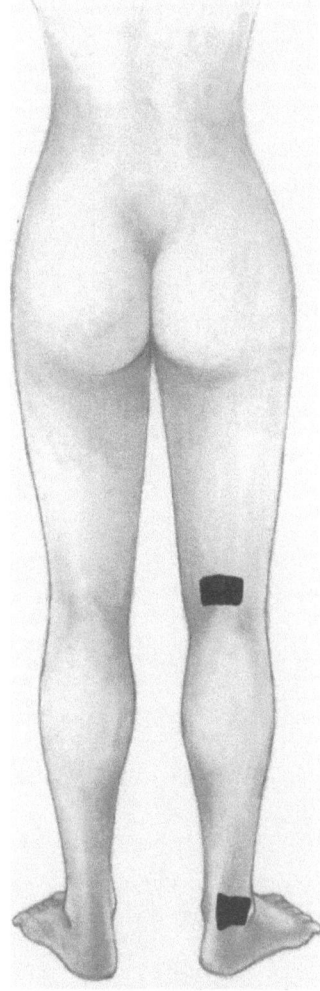 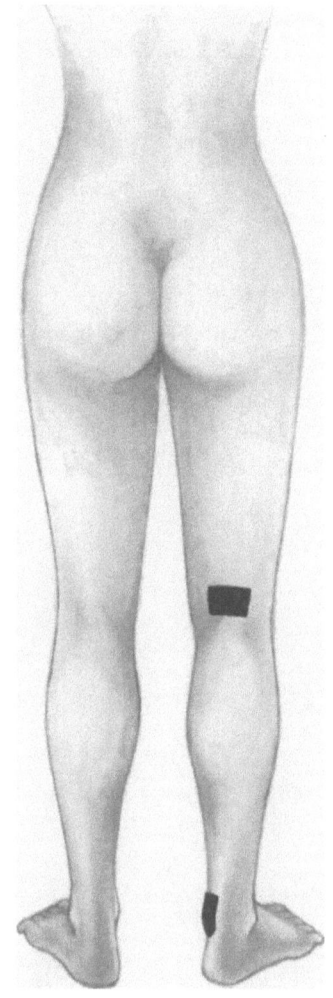

Fig. 3.40                                        Fig. 3.41

Fig. 3.40. Lateral ischaemic pain in the foot. *Electrode placement sites:* popliteal crease and in depression between lateral malleous and tendo-achilles. *Recommended mode of stimulation:* high frequency or low-frequency trains, intensity just below pain threshold. *Polarity:* Generally of no importance

Fig. 3.41. Medial ischaemic pain in the foot. *Electrode placement sites:* Dorsal web space and volar surface of wrist/hand. *Recommended mode of stimulation:* Low-frequency pulse-trains, high intensity. *Polarity:* the negative electrode should be positioned on the dorsal web space

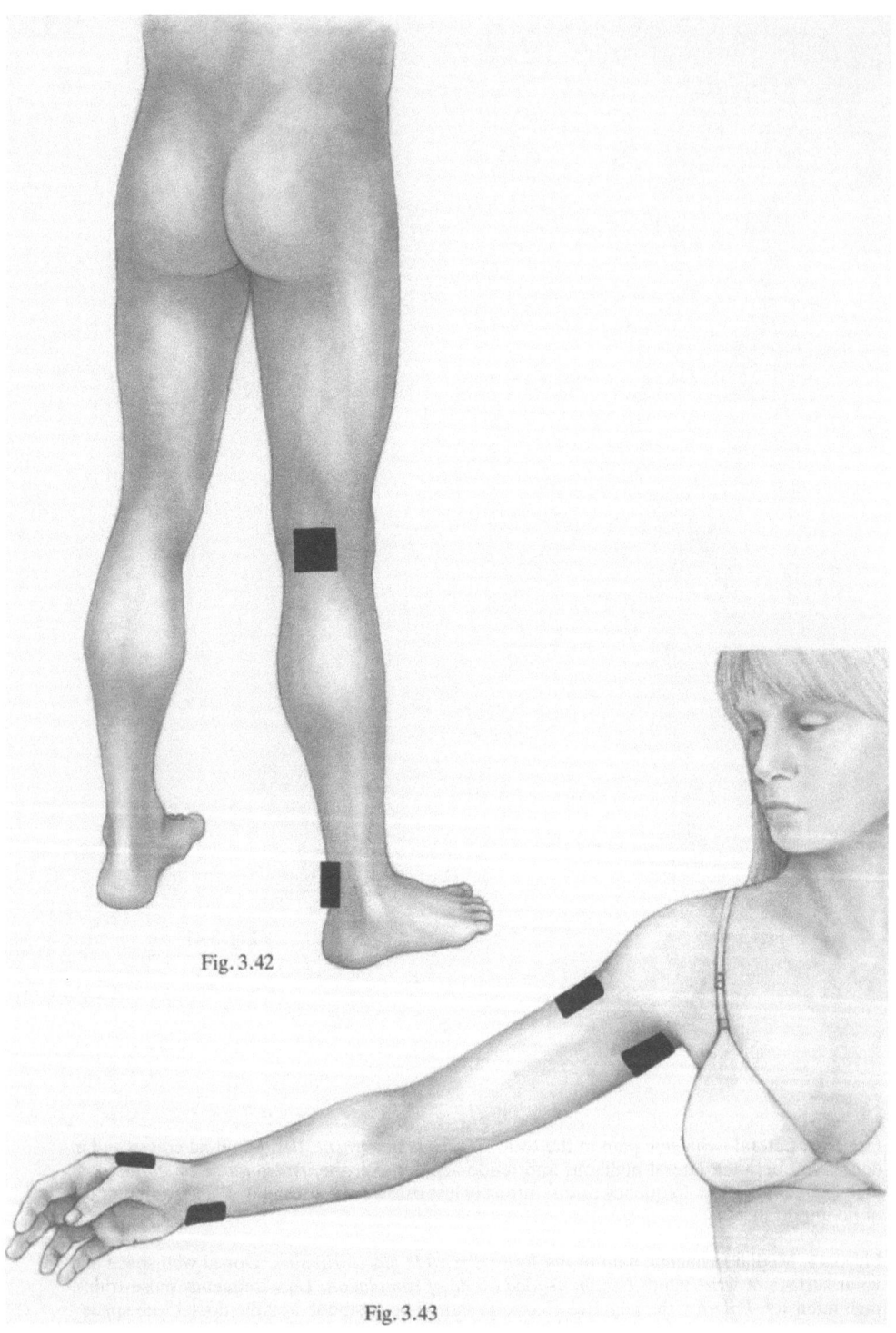

Fig. 3.42

Fig. 3.43

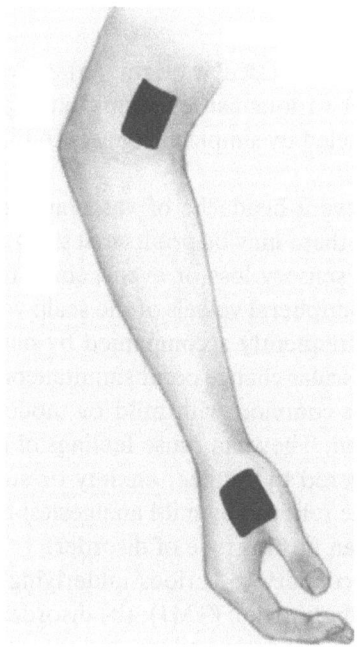

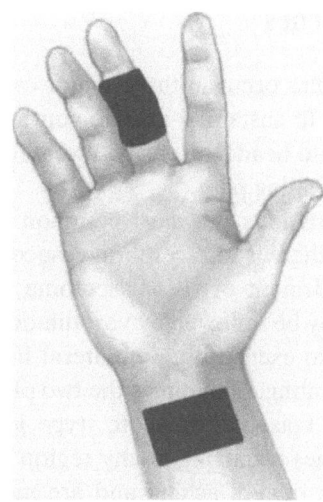

Fig. 3.45

Fig. 3.44

Fig. 3.42. Thromboplebitis (saphenous vein) pain in the right leg. *Electrode placement sites:* popliteal crease and in depression between medial malleolus and tendo Achillis. *Recommended mode of stimulation:* high frequency or low-frequency trains, intensity below pain threshold. *Polarity:* generally of no importance

Fig. 3.43. Raynaud's phenomenon. *Electrode placement sites:* one pair at dorsal web space and posterolateral to deltoid insertion; another pair at lower axilla, medial to brachial artery and volar surface of wrist. *Recommended mode of stimulation:* high frequency or low-frequency trains, intensity just below pain threshold. *Polarity:* generally of no importance

Fig. 3.44. Alternative electrode placements in Raynaud's phenomenon. *Electrode placement sites:* dorsal web space and in depression at lateral end of elbow crease. *Recommended mode of stimulation:* high frequency or low-frequency trains, intensity just below pain threshold. *Polarity:* generally of no importance

Fig. 3.45. Vascular insult to middle finger. *Electrode placement sites:* volar aspect of wrist and proximal to distal phalanx around volar surface of second finger. *Recommended mode of stimulation:* low-frequency trains, producing rhythmical contractions. *Polarity:* generally of no importance

# Headaches

Headaches occur in three major categories: (a) of vascular origin; (b) episodic; (c) due to sustained muscle contraction with various causes. Symptoms range from mild headache easily tolerated or controlled by simple analgesics to totally incapacitating pain.

Migraine is the most common type of severe headache of vascular origin. Where there is intracerebral vasoconstriction there may be prodromal signs such as impairment of vision, scotoma, transient sensory loss or even hemiparesis. This may be followed by vasodilation of the peripheral vessels of the scalp which results in excruciating unilateral headache, frequently accompanied by nausea and vomiting. Sometimes the two phases of vascular change occur simultaneously.

The episodic, or acute, type is the most common with mild or moderate headaches occurring in any region of the head. They can cause feelings of constriction or dull aching and are mostly triggered by fatigue, anxiety or stress. They usually subside following rest or may be relieved by mild analgesics; most sufferers do not need to consult their physician for this type of disorder.

Muscle contraction headaches may be secondary to various underlying disorders such as: (a) temperomandibular joint dysfunction (TMJ); (b) disorders of the cervical spine (degenerative arthritis, ankylosing spondylosis and discogenic disease); (c) trauma (post-concussion, whiplash injuries); (d) nasal or paranasal inflammation; (e) inflammation secondary to systemic disorders (viral infections). The chronic variety presents a difficult pain management problem. The characteristics are often similar to those in the episodic type, but the pain is unremitting and may be present for weeks, months or years. Tension, anxiety and depression are apt to occur along with chronic headaches. Treatment of chronic muscle contraction headache consists of first weaning the patient away from the use of regular large-scale analgesic medication which may have perpetuated the chronicity of the pain. A strong effort should be made by the physician to have patients discontinue this abuse.

## Usefulness of TENS in Headaches

Reports in the literature pertaining specifically to the use of TENS in headaches are sparse. Shealy (1976) recommends placement of electrodes over the occipital nerves with an intensity of stimulation high enough to produce paraesthesia from occiput to vertex. If this is not successful, stimulation over the forehead or temples is recommended. The effectiveness of TENS in the relief of headaches is dependent on how long the headache has existed. The best results have been obtained when stimulation is initiated at or close to the onset of the headache. Omura (1981) has reported good results with the use of TENS in the treatment of headaches classified as cephalic hypertension or hypotension. During treatment the two electrodes were placed suboccipitally or on the trapezius. The patients were treated for 20 min with a strong, low-rate (1 or 2 Hz) mode.

Shealy (1976) and Mannheimer and Lampe (1984) have reported that TENS may be used with satisfactory results for treatment of headache in connection with temperomandibular joint dysfunction.

## References

Mannheimer JS, Lampe GN (1984) Clinical transcutaneous electrical nerve stimulation. Davis, Philadelphia
Omura Y (1981) Simple custom made disposable surface electrode system for non-invasive "electro-acupuncture" or TNS and its clinical applications including treatment of cephalic-hypertension and hypotension syndromes as well as temperomandibular joint problems, tinnitus, shoulder and lower back pain, etc. Acupunct Electrother Res 6:109
Shealy CN (1976) The pain game. Celestial Arts, Millbrae, CA, p 80

## Suggested Reading

Bates JAV, Nathan PW (1980) Transcutaneous electrical nerve stimulation for chronic pain. Anaesthesia 35:817
Cauthen JC, Renner EJ (1975) Transcutaneous and peripheral nerve stimulation for chronic pain states. Surg Neurol 4:102
Eriksson MBE, Sjölund BH (1978) Pain relief from conventional versus acupuncturelike-TNS in patients with chronic facial pain. In: Pain abstracts. Second World Congress on Pain, IASP, Montreal, p 128
Ignelzi RJ, Sternbach RA, Callaghan M (1979) Somatosensory changes during transcutaneous electrical analgesia. In: Bonica JJ, Albe-Fessard D (eds) Advances in pain research and therapy, vol 1. Raven, New York, p 509
Kirsch WM, Lewis JA, Simon RH (1975) Experiences with electrical stimulation devices for the control of chronic pain. Med Instrum 9:217
Laitinen L (1976) Placement of electrodes in transcutaneous stimulation for chronic pain. Neurochirurgie 22:517
Loeser JD, Black RG, Christman (1975) Relief of pain by transcutaneous stimulation. J Neurosurg 42:308
McKelvy P (1978) Clinical report on the use of specific TENS units. Phys Ther 58:1474
Picaza JA et al (1975) Pain suppression by peripheral nerve stimulation. I Observation with transcutaneous stimuli. Surg Neurol 4:105
Shealy CN (1974) Electrical control of the nervous system. Med Prog Technol 2:71
Shealy CN, Kwako JL, Hughes S (1979) Effects of transcranial neurostimulation upon mood and serotonin production: a preliminary report. Il Dolore 1:13
Tichou-Olshwang D, Magora F (1980) Relief of pain by subcutaneous electrical nerve stimulation after ocular surgery. Am J Ophthalmol 89:903

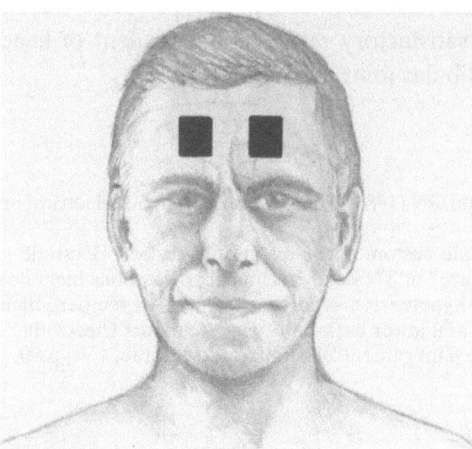

Fig. 3.46. Bilateral frontal headache. *Electrode placement sites:* supraorbitally. *Recommended mode of stimulation:* high frequency or low-frequency trains, intensity just below pain threshold. *Polarity:* generally of no importance

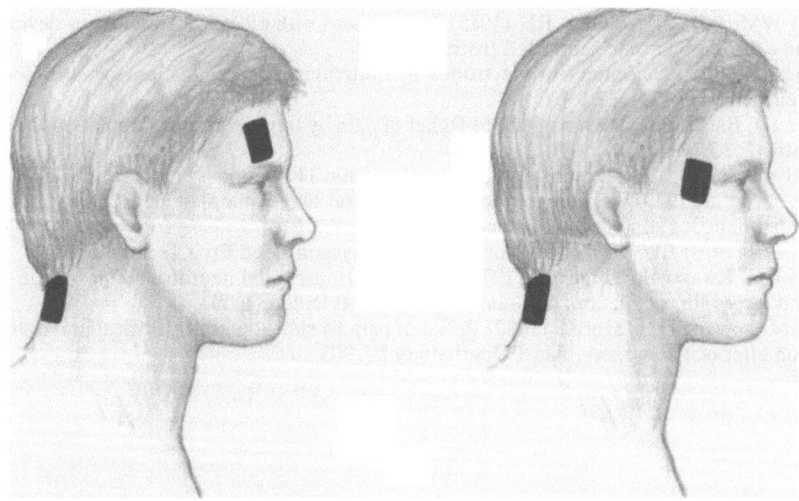

Fig. 3.47                                    Fig. 3.48

Fig. 3.47. Unilateral frontal headache. *Electrode placement sites:* supraorbitally and suboccipitally. *Recommended mode of stimulation:* high frequency or low-frequency trains, intensity just below pain threshold. *Polarity:* generally of no importance

Fig. 3.48. Temporal headache. *Electrode placement sites:* temporal fossa, lateral to eyebrow and suboccipitally. *Recommended mode of stimulation:* high frequency or low-frequency trains, intensity just below pain threshold. *Polarity:* generally of no importance

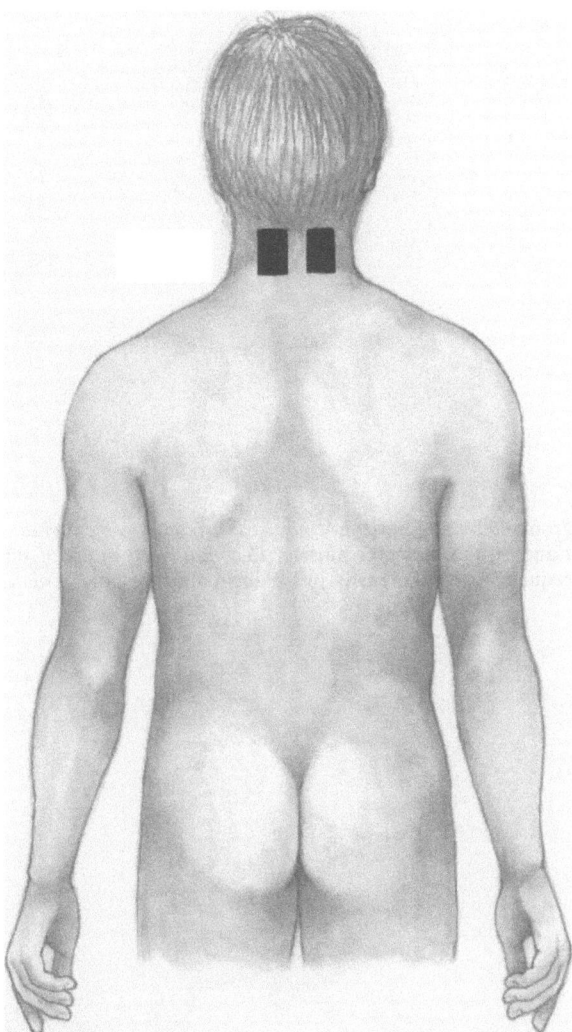

Fig. 3.49. Bifrontal headache due to cervical strain. *Electrode placement sites:* suboccipitally and bilaterally. *Recommended mode of stimulation:* high frequency or low-frequency trains, intensity just below pain threshold. *Polarity:* generally of no importance

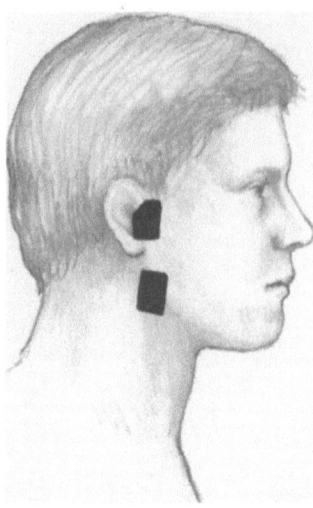

Fig. 3.50. Temperomandibular joint syndrome. *Electrode placement sites:* over the tempero-mandibular joint and on the masseter muscle. *Recommended mode of stimulation:* high fre-quency or low-frequency train, intensity just below pain threshold. *Polarity:* generally of no importance

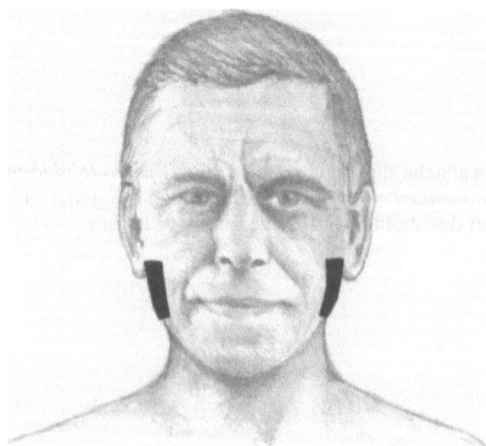

Fig. 3.51. Temperomandibular joint syndrome. *Electrode placement sites:* over each tempero-mandibular joint (upper region of masseter muscle). *Recommended mode of stimulation:* low-frequency trains, producing rhythmical contractions. *Polarity:* generally of no importance

# Dental Pain

The most common pain in the orofacial region originates from the teeth and their supporting structures, i.e. the peridontium. Generally, dental pain is a sequela of dental caries. Initially, when the carious lesion is restricted to the dentine, there is no spontaneous pain. However, as the caries penetrates deeper into tooth and pulp, inflammatory processes commence associated with intermittent spontaneous pain. Constant pain is seen if the inflammatory processes invade the area around the tooth root apex (periodontitis).

## Usefulness of TENS in Dental Pain

TENS can be applied for control of acute dental pain. Hansson ånd Ekblom (1983) evaluated 62 patients admitted to an emergency dental clinic with acute pain secondary to pulpal inflammation, apical periodontitis, or post-operative pain after tooth extraction. Patients were randomly divided into three groups: those receiving high-frequency TENS, those receiving low-frequency train TENS and those receiving placebo. The results show that high-frequency and low-frequency train TENS were equally effective and significantly more so than placebo.

In a study by Roth and Trash (1986) TENS was assessed for its effect on periodontal pain associated with orthodontic separation. Forty-five patients were randomly allocated to a TENS group, a placebo TENS group and a control group. They were further subdivided into intraoral and extraoral electrode

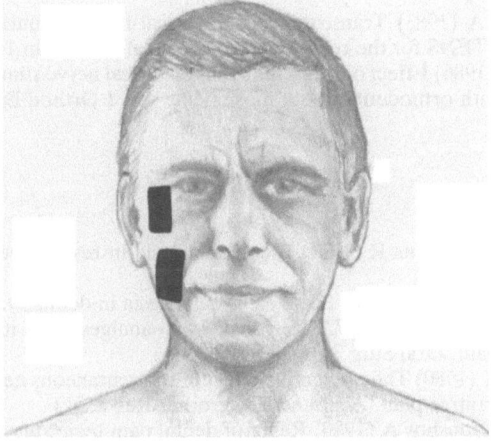

Fig. 3.52. Dental pain in the upper jaw. *Electrode placement sites:* over temperomandibular joint and on masseter muscle. *Recommended mode of stimulation:* high frequency, intensity just below pain threshold. *Polarity:* generally of no importance

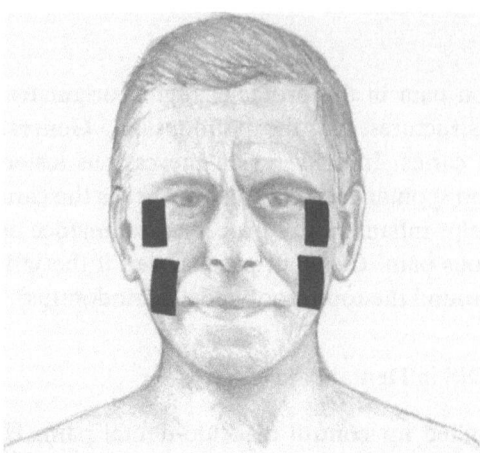

Fig. 3.53. Diffuse dental pain. *Electrode placement sites:* over temperomandibular joint and on masseter muscle bilaterally. *Recommended mode of stimulation:* high frequency or low-frequency trains, intensity just below pain threshold. *Polarity:* generally of no importance

placement, and 1–3-day treatment duration groups. In each patient orthodontic separators were placed bilaterally mesial and distal to the upper first molars. Subjects were asked to rate their discomfort (pain) every 12 h for 4 days. The results showed a significant decrease in reported pain for the subjects in the TENS group at 24-, 36- and 48-h assessment periods compared to those in either the placebo or control group. In the control group post-separation discomfort continued through the 60-h assessment period.

### References

Hansson P, Ekblom A (1983) Transcutaneous electrical nerve stimulation (TENS) as compared to placebo TENS for the relief of acute orofacial pain. Pain 15:157
Roth PM, Trash WJ (1986) Effect of transcutaneous electrical nerve stimulation for controlling pain associated with orthodontic tooth movement. Am J Orthod Dentofacial Orthop 90: 132

### Suggested Reading

Bradley JF, Brooks B, Umans R (1974) Electroanalgesia in restorative dentistry. J Prosthet Dent 32:171
Brooks B, Reiss R, Umans R (1970) Local electroanalgesia in dentistry. J Dent Res 49:298
Fields RW, Savara BS, Tocke R (1972) Regional electroanalgesia and its potentialities in control of orofacial pain. Oral Surg 34:694
Ihalainen V, Perkki K (1980) The preventive effect of transcutaneous nerve stimulation (TNS) on acute post-operative pain. Acupunct Electrother Res 5:313
Melzack R, Guite S, Gonshor A (1980) Relief of dental pain by ice massage of the hand. Can Med Assoc J 122:189
Shealy CN (1974) Electrical control of the nervous system. Med Prog Technol 2:71
Strassburg HM, Krainick JV, Thoden V (1977) Influence of transcutaneous nerve stimulation (TNS) on acute pain. J Neurol 217:1

# Cancer Pain

Cancer may cause pain in a wide variety of ways. Also, each type of malignant pain may be described by patients in different terms and aggravated or relieved by different factors. Therefore, each cancer pain patient requires a personal therapeutic approach. In recent years a great deal of clinical and research work has been put into the treatment of malignant pain. It has been shown that the control of cancer pain may be improved and drug side effects reduced if an exact diagnosis of the cause(s) of the pain is made and an appropriate treatment given. Such treatment involves analgesics and non-pharmacological methods such as nerve blocks and TENS.

## Usefulness of TENS in Cancer Pain

Clinical studies have documented the successful one of TENS in various types of cancer pain. Ventafridda et al. (1979) used TENS in 37 patients with intractable pain due to cancer. During the first 10 days, TENS was successful in markedly reducing pain in 96% of the patients, but the rate declined dramatically. After 30 days, only four patients (11%) continued to obtain pain relief. The use of analgesics, however, was reduced in 54% of the patients even after 1 month of TENS.

## Reference

Ventafridda V et al (1979) Transcutaneous nerve stimulation in cancer pain. In: Bonica JJ, Ventafridda V (eds) Advances in pain research and therapy, vol 2. Raven, New York, p 509

## Suggested Reading

Kirsch WM, Lewis JA, Simon RH (1975) Experiences with electrical stimulation devices for the control of chronic pain. Med Instrum 9:217
Loeser JD, Black RG, Christman A (1975) Relief of pain by transcutaneous stimulation. J Neurosurg 42:308
Long DM (1976) Cutaneous afferent stimulation for the relief of pain. Prog Neurol Surg 7:35
Ostrowski MJ, Dodd VA (1977) Transcutaneous nerve stimulation for relief of pain in advanced malignant disease. Nurs Times Aug 11, p 1233
Picaza JA et al (1975) Pain suppression by peripheral nerve stimulation. I. Observation with transcutaneous stimuli. Surg Neurol 4:105
Shealy CN (1974) Electrical control of the nervous system. Med Prog Technol 2:71

# Dysmenorrhea

Dysmenorrhea is a common complaint in about 10% of females in their late teens and early twenties. Pain is often so severe that the woman has to stay in bed for 1–2 days, thereby occasioning frequent absences from work. The evidence indicates that prostaglandins regulate myometrial contractility which leads to ischaemia. This may be the underlying cause of primary dysmenorrhea. Interestingly, elevated levels of $F_2$ prostaglandins and metabolites have been found in the menstrual fluid of dysmenorrheic women and the levels of these in endometrium and plasma seem to correlate very well to the incidence of pain. It has been reported that the degree of potency of analgesics in alleviating dysmenorrhea is related to their effectiveness in depressing prostaglandin synthesis or its action. Also, calcium-antagonistic agents such as nifedipine and verapamil have been shown to reduce prostaglandin-induced uterine hypercontractility, thereby relieving menstrual pain. Other drugs which have been used in the treatment of primary dysmenorrhea are hormonal preparations (estrogen) which inhibit ovulation. A non-pharmacological method for the alleviation of dysmenorrhea can be of great value especially in patients suffering various side effects from drugs used.

## Usefulness of TENS in Dysmenorrhea

In a study by Mannheimer and Lampe (1984) the effect of TENS was examined in a group of female college students. Twenty-seven subjects with a history of menstrual pain and not on oral contraceptives were randomly assigned to one of three groups: control, high-frequency TENS and strong low-frequency TENS. Results showed a mean decrease in pain of 72% using high-frequency TENS, 52% using low-frequency TENS and 26% using the control TENS. High-frequency TENS produced a mean duration of pain relief of 4.2 h compared to 2.5 h in the low-frequency group. Furthermore, participants in the high-frequency TENS group were able to pursue their usual activities during stimulation, and 70% of the subjects wished to continue its use.

　　Heltzel et al. (1987) studied the effect of TENS in 14 patients with severe dysmenorrhea of several years' duration. Significant reductions in cramping, low back pain and analgesic intake were demonstrated in all patients using a three-electrode placement forming an inverted triangular pattern about the umbilicus.

　　Lundeberg et al. (1985) have reported on the use of high-frequency TENS, low-frequency train TENS or placebo TENS in 21 patients suffering from primary dysmenorrhea. The results show that 14 out of 21 patients receiving high-frequency TENS experienced a pain reduction exceeding 50%. During low-frequency TENS and placebo TENS, seven and five patients, respectively, obtained pain relief exceeding 50%.

# References

Heltzel JA, Senta TA, Weeks ME (1987) Effective control of primary dysmenorrhea pain using transcutaneous electrical nerve stimulation (TENS). Pain [Suppl] 4:370

Lundeberg T, Bondesson L, Lundström V (1985) Relief of primary dysmenorrhea by transcutaneous electrical nerve stimulation. Acta Obstet Gynecol Scand 64:491–497

Mannheimer JS, Lampe GN (1984) Clinical transcutaneous electrical nerve stimulation. Davis, Philadelphia

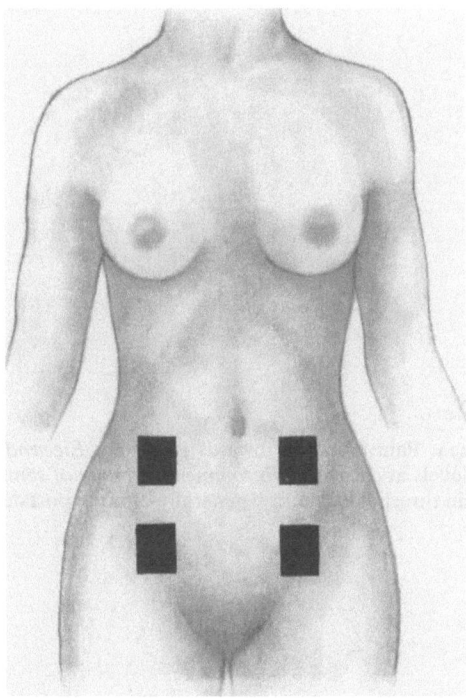

Fig. 3.54. Dysmenorrhea. Pain radiating ventrally, mainly in the suprapubic region. *Electrode placement sites:* one pair on abdomen in anterolateral area of pain below umbilicus on right and left side; another pain on abdomen above anterior-superior iliac spine on right and left side. *Recommended mode of stimulation:* high frequency, intensity just below pain threshold. *Polarity:* generally of no importance

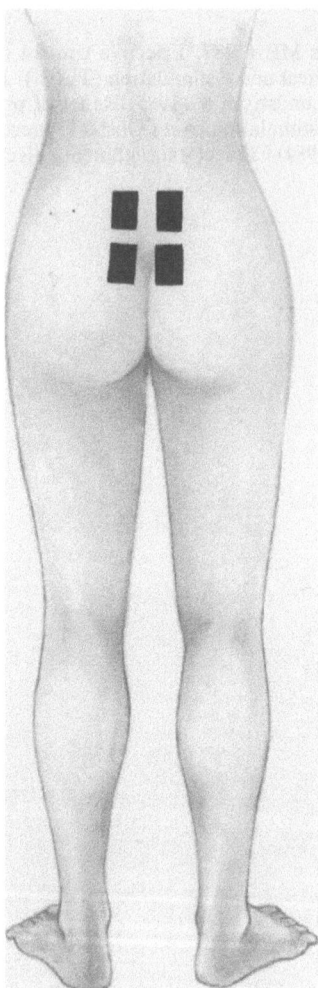

Fig. 3.55. Dysmenorrhea. Pain radiating towards the back. *Electrode placement sites:* para-spinally at L3 and S2 levels at each side. *Recommended mode of stimulation:* high frequency, intensity just below pain threshold. *Polarity:* generally of no importance

# Labour Pain

Labour pain and pain during pregnancy have always been two of the most important issues of the health care system of many countries. Despite recent evidence that properly administered anaesthesia provides relief and reduces perinatal mortality many women still suffer severe pain during parturition.

## Usefulness of TENS in Pregnancy and Parturition

TENS has been used successfully to control pain during labour and delivery (Jones 1980). The recommended electrode placement has been two electrode pairs paraspinally: one electrode pair at T10–L1 for the first stage of labour and one pair at S2–S4 for the second stage of labour. In a study by Augustinsson et al. (1977) on 147 women during labour, 48% obtained good to very good pain control, 37% obtained moderate relief and 15% had no benefit. Shealy and Maurer (1974) reported excellent relief of back pain during parturition in most patients studied, but only three out of 50 obtained satisfactory relief of anterior pain. They reported that anterior pain can be relieved by placement of electrodes on the abdomen or groin.

Bundsen and Ericson (1982) have conducted extensive studies on the use of TENS during labour and delivery. They have found no harmful effects to mother or foetus with low back stimulation. In the patients with suprapubic pain, Bundsen and Ericson (1982) recommend suprapubic electrode placement.

Erkola et al. (1980) evaluated 100 patients who used TENS for pain management during the first stage of labour. Electrodes were placed paravertebrally at T10-11 and S2-4. Stimulus intensity was set at a non-painful level and regulated by the patient. Good pain relief was reported by 31% of the patients, and 55% reported moderate relief within 1 h of initiating treatment. Grim and Morey (1985) reported on 15 patients who served as their own control and turned the unit off for several contractions during the middle and late periods of the first stage of labour to judge the effectiveness of TENS. Nearly all of the women reported some relief during labour and excellent relief was reported by three. Most participants expressed a willingness to use TENS for future deliveries.

Tischendorf (1986) studied 78 women who used TENS for labour pains. TENS electrodes were placed at T10-L2 without electrostimulation of the sacral segments. TENS produced a marked reduction in duration of labour. Also, using TENS clearly reduced the amounts of spasmolytic agents that had to be administered during labour.

Harrison et al. (1986) have also reported on TENS in pain relief during labour. The analgesic effect of TENS in labour was investigated in a double-blind TENS/placebo TENS controlled trial in 100 primigravidae and 50 women in their third labour. There were no differences between the TENS and the placebo TENS users in terms of pain or relief, and only two women completed

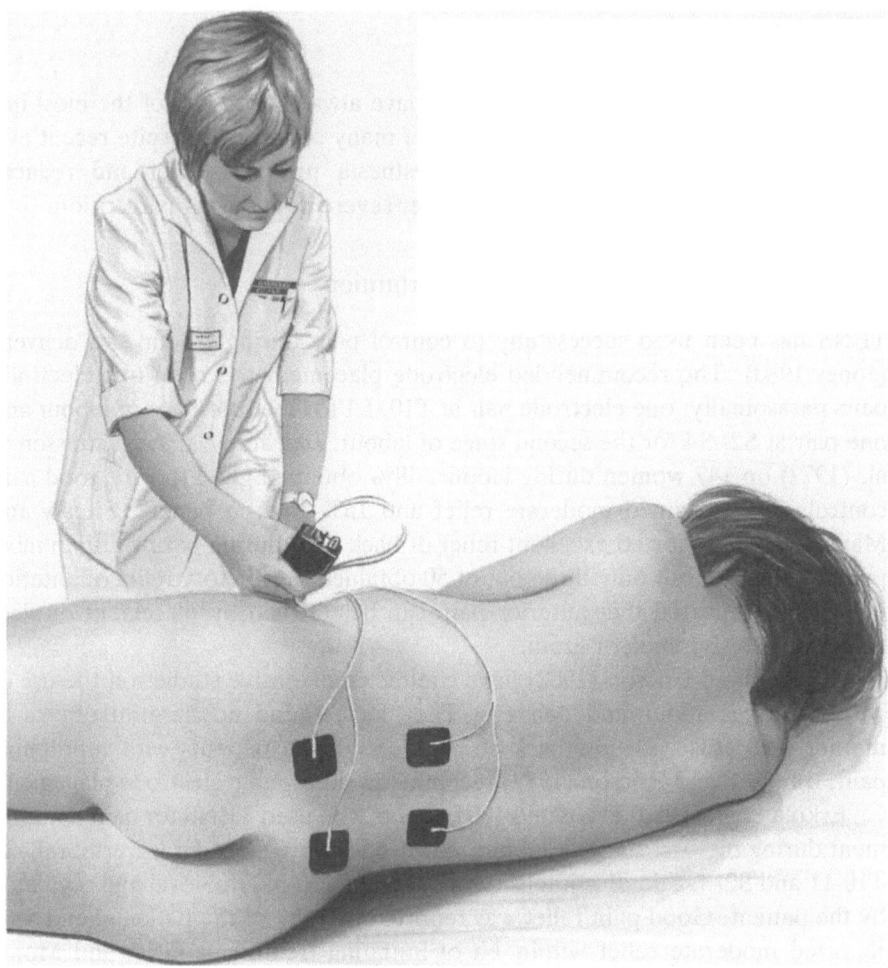

Fig. 3.56. Labour pain. *Electrode placement sites:* paraspinally on left and right side at T10–L1 level and S2–S4 level. *Recommended mode of stimulation:* high frequency, intensity just below pain threshold. *Polarity:* generally of no importance

labour without requiring other additional analgesia. The primigravidae who used either TENS or placebo TENS alone had shorter labours than those who required further analgesia.

Getland and Jeans (1986) have reported on post-operative pain of 18 multiparous women who had all undergone elective Caesarean delivery. Nine patients received TENS and nine placebo stimulation. The treatment was continuous through to the 3rd day following the day of surgery. The results suggest that TENS was significantly more effective than placebo TENS in reducing cutaneous, movement-associated incisional pain. However, pain resulting from internal structures, i.e. deep pain, afterbirth pain (due to uterine contractions) and the somatic pain associated with decreased peristalsis (gas pains) were not amenable to TENS. No significant differences in analgesic intake were observed.

## References

Augustinsson LE et al (1977) Pain relief during delivery by transcutaneous electrical nerve stimulation. Pain 4:59

Bundsen P, Ericson K (1982) Pain relief in labour by transcutaneous electrical nerve stimulation: safety aspects. Acta Obstet Gynecol Scand 61:1

Erkola R, Pikkola P, Kanto J (1980) Transcutaneous nerve stimulation for pain relief during labour: a controlled study. Ann Chir Gynaecol 69:273

Getland MM, Jeans ME (1986) The effects of transcutaneous electrical nerve stimulation on post-cesarean pain. Pain 27:181

Grim LC, Morey SH (1985) Transcutaneous electrical nerve stimulation for relief of parturition pain. A clinical report. Phys Ther 65:337

Harrison RF, Woods T, Shore M, Mathews G, Unwin A (1986) Pain relief in labour using transcutaneous electrical nerve stimulation (TENS). A TENS/TENS placebo controlled study two parity groups. Br J Obstet Gynaecol 93:739

Jones MCMH (1980) Transcutaneous nerve stimulation in labour. Anaesthesia 35:372

Shealy CN, Maurer D (1974) Transcutaneous nerve stimulation for control of pain: a preliminary technical note. Surg Neurol 2:45

Tischendorf D (1986) Die transkutane elektrische Nervenstimulation (TENS) in der Geburtshilfe. Zentralbl Gynakol 108:486

## Suggested Reading

Kubista E, Kucera H, Riss P (1978) The effect of transcutaneous nerve stimulation on labour pain. Geburtshilfe Frauenheilkd 38:1079

Neumark J, Pauser G, Schirzer W (1978) Pain relief in childbirth: an analysis of the analgesic effects of transcutaneous nerve stimulation (TNS), pethidine and placebos. Prak Anaesth 13:13

# Bladder Pain

In the field of visceral pain, bladder pain has attracted much interest due to its complex pathophysiology. Despite recent advances in medicine, the proper management of patients with bladder pain remains to be solved.

## Usefulness of TENS in Bladder Pain

Beneficial effects have been reported with TENS in patients with bladder pain and frequent micturition. In a study by Fall et al. (1980) on patients who had previously been treated unsuccessfully by conservative means, TENS was applied suprapubically with the electrodes 10–15 cm apart. TENS was carried out for 15 min–2 h per day at the maximally tolerated level. All patients showed slight increases in bladder volume, voiding frequency decreased, and pain was reduced. Bladder lesions significantly decreased over a 6-month period.

Leyson et al. (1979) studied the effects of TENS on bladder and sphincter function in a group of 17 patients with acute and chronic spinal cord injuries. TENS was applied to the C4–6, T10, L5 and S2 dermatomes. Treatments were given for 20–30 min daily for at least 30 days and were continued if satisfactory pain relief occurred. TENS applied in the L5 and S2 dermatomes affected the urodynamic function, and TENS at segments above the T10 level resulted in an increase of residual urine volumes. Also, Piancentini et al. (1986) have reported that TENS may inhibit the detrusor activity in patients with a neurogenic bladder.

## References

Fall M, Carlsson CA, Erlandson BE (1980) Electrical stimulation in interstitial cystitis. J Urol 123:192
Leyson JFJ, Stefaniwsky L, Martin BF (1979) Effects of transcutaneous nerve stimulation on the vesicourethral function in spinal cord injury patients. J Urol 121:635
Piancentini F, Prati R, Gandellini G, Prati A (1986) Influenze della stimolazione transcutanea (TENS) del tibiale posteriore su alcuni parametri cista monometrici in pazienti con vesica neurologica. Primi dati su sei pazienti. Acta Biomed Ateneo Parmenese 57:109–113

# Pancreatic Pain

Acute pancreatitis is characterised by severe abdominal pain, generalised or in the upper quadrants and radiating to the back. It increases steadily, reaches a maximum in a few minutes or hours and then usually remains severe and unrelenting until it diminishes gradually over days or weeks as the inflammation subsides. In chronic pancreatitis the pain may be persistent or intermittent. It is usually localised to the upper abdomen or may be generalised, commonly radiating to the back. It may be described as aching, burning, gnawing or stabbing and is usually present for weeks.

Usefulness of TENS in Pancreatic Pain

There are few reports on the use of TENS in pancreatic pain. Roberts (1978) used TENS to manage pancreatic pain in five patients. Electrodes were placed on the upper abdomen or epigastrium. Stimulation was performed two to six times for 30–60 min at intervals of 1–3 days. High-frequency TENS was used, but brief, intense stimulation was occasionally employed to initially break through persistent pain. All five patients had prompt and lasting relief of upper abdominal pain after two treatments. Subsequent painful episodes were managed with TENS, and hospitalisation was not required. However, Ballegaard et al. (1985) have reported that out of 23 patients with pancreatitis, neither electroacupuncture nor TENS brought about pain relief that could supplement or substitute medical treatment.

## References

Ballegaard S, Christophersen SJ, Dawids SG, Hesse J, Olsen NV (1985) Acupuncture and transcutaneous electrical nerve stimulation in the treatment of pain associated with chronic pancreatitis. A randomized study. Scand J Gastroenterol 20:1249
Roberts HJ (1978) Transcutaneous electrical nerve stimulation in the management of pancreatitis pain. South Med J 71:396

# Psychogenic Pain

It is a well-known fact that emotional stress may trigger pain or reintroduce old pain in the absence of pathological organic states. A number of investigators have proposed a "pain-anxiety-tension" cycle to account for some forms of acute and chronic psychogenic pain. This vicious circle has been observed frequently in disorders involving the musculoskeletal system.

Usefulness of TENS in Psychogenic Pain

Several authors have reported that patients with psychogenic pain generally do not respond well to TENS (Long and Hagfors 1975; Eriksson et al. 1979). In a study by Lehmann et al. (1983) 54 patients treated in a 3-week inpatient rehabilitation programme were randomly assigned to electro-acupuncture, high-frequency TENS or placebo TENS. Two groups were formed based on the absence of non-organic physical findings (valid group) and on the presence of two or more non-organic physical findings (invalid group). Statistical analyses were utilised to determine the effects of the treatment and the effects of over-reporting (presence of excessive non-organic physical findings). Interestingly, a number of the patients reported an increase of pain with TENS. Statistically significant findings demonstrated that the acupuncture group enjoyed more relief of peak pain and more relief of pain on an average day at the 3-month return assessment. Additionally, the acupuncture group demonstrated greater improvement in extension trunk strength at the discharge assessment.

## References

Eriksson MBE, Sjölund BH, Neilzen S (1979) Long term results of peripheral conditioning stimulation as analgesic measure in chronic pain. Pain 6:335
Lehmann TR, Russell DW, Spratt KF (1983) The impact of patients with non-organic physical findings on a controlled trial of transcutaneous electrical nerve stimulation and electro-acupuncture. Spine 8:625–634
Long DM, Hagfors N (1975) Electrical stimulation of the nervous system: the current status of electrical stimulation of the nervous system for relief of pain. Pain 1:109

## Suggested Reading

Long DM (1977) Cutaneous afferent stimulation for the relief of pain. Prog Neurol Surg 7:35
Long DM (1977) The comparative efficacy of drugs vs electrical modulation in the management of chronic pain. In: Le Roy PL (ed) Current concepts in the management of chronic pain. Symposia Specialists, Miami, p 53

# Chapter 4  Additional Areas of Application of TENS and Different Modes of Electrical Stimulation

New alternatives for the use of electrical currents have grown out of an increasing understanding of the effects of electrical stimulation on various physiological functions. Except for pain treatment, electrical stimulation has been frequently used for improvement of muscle functions and for the treatment of circulatory disorders. A variety of stimulation techniques have been used including TENS and other stimulus parameters. For a detailed description of the techniques used in these studies the reader is referred to the original articles.

## Sports Medicine

In past years there has been a growing interest in the use of TENS in sports medicine. TENS has in general been used in combination with other modes of treatment to facilitate an effective rehabilitation programme. Preliminary studies have also shown that TENS may be used to improve physical performance.

### Usefulness of TENS in Sports Injuries and Physical Performance

Jensen et al. (1986) have reported that TENS relieves pain following shoulder dislocations and acromioclavicular joint subluxations. These authors also treated traumatic contusions of the iliac crest, tennis elbows, ankle sprains and cervical and lumbar sprains with good results. They conclude that TENS should not be used in situations of physical stress to increase endurance, since pain in these situations serves as a warning against overstress. However, after periods of physical activity TENS may be useful for relieving muscle ache and fatigue.

In a pilot study Kaada (1984) tested the physical performance in 21 athletes who received low-frequency TENS for 30–45 min prior to a road or track race, swimming race, bicycle ergometer exercise, isometric muscular endurance tests or dynamometer hand grip test. Improved performance was seen compared with controls without TENS or with placebo stimulation in the same subjects and was observed in running, swimming and ergometer cycling, although with great individual variations.

References

Jensen JE, Etheridge GL, Hazelrigg G (1986) Effectiveness of transcutaneous electrical neural stimulation in the treatment of pain. Recommendations for use in the treatment of sports injuries. Sports Med 3:79
Kaada B (1984) Improvement of physical performance by transcutaneous nerve stimulation in athletes. Acupunct Electrother Res 9:165

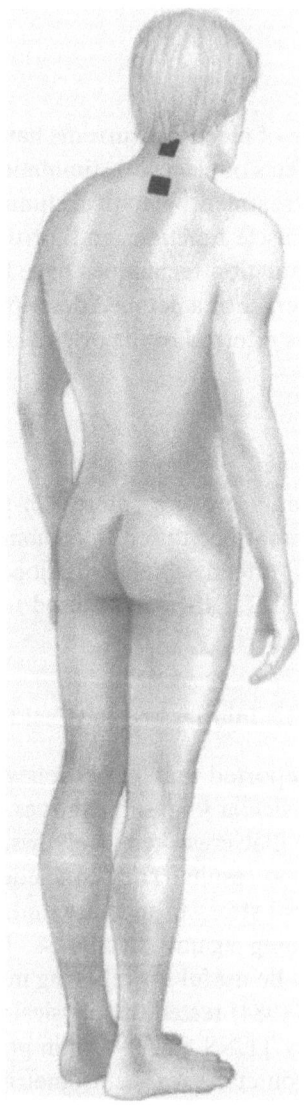

Fig. 4.1. Cervical strain. *Electrode placement sites:* suboccipitally and in superior medial angle of scapula. *Recommended mode of stimulation:* high frequency or low-frequency trains, intensity just below pain threshold. *Polarity:* it is recommended that the cathode is connected to the electrode placed at the superior medial angle of scapula. However, generally of no importance

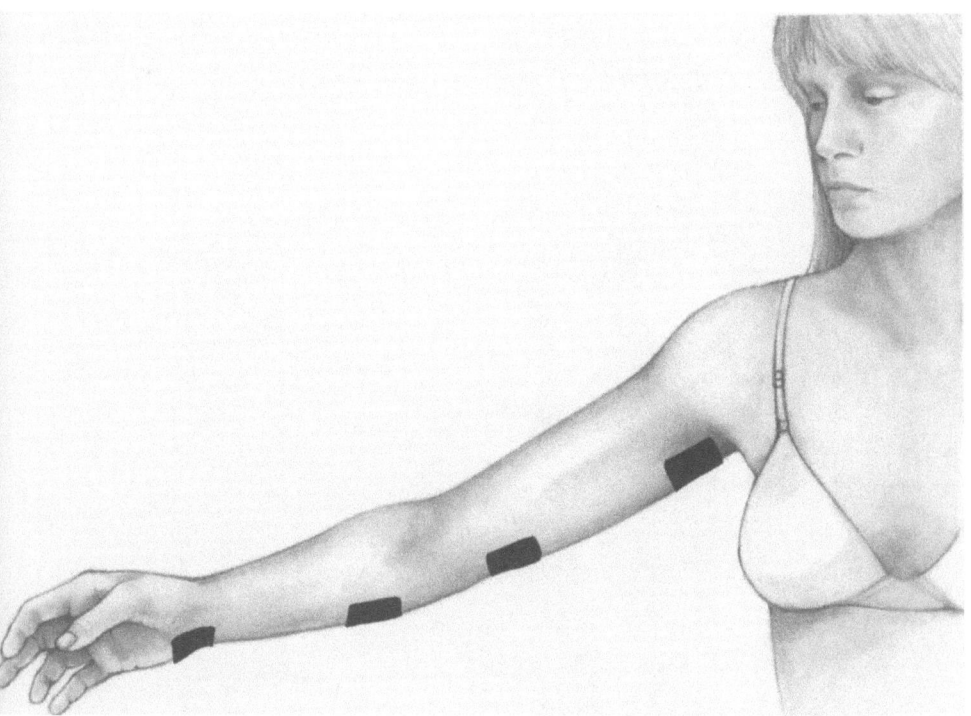

Fig. 4.2. Cervical trauma with cervico-brachialgia in the C8 segment. *Electrode placement sites:* one pair at lower axilla and below olecranon groove; another pair at volar surface of distal forearm and ulnar border of wrist. *Recommended mode of stimulation:* high frequency or low-frequency trains, intensity just below pain threshold. *Polarity:* high frequency if skin sensitivity is normal. The cathodes should be connected to the electrode at the lower axilla and volar surface of the distal forearm. The anodes should be connected to the electrodes below the olecranon groove and ulnar border of wrist. In case of sensitivity loss, the reversed polarity is recommended

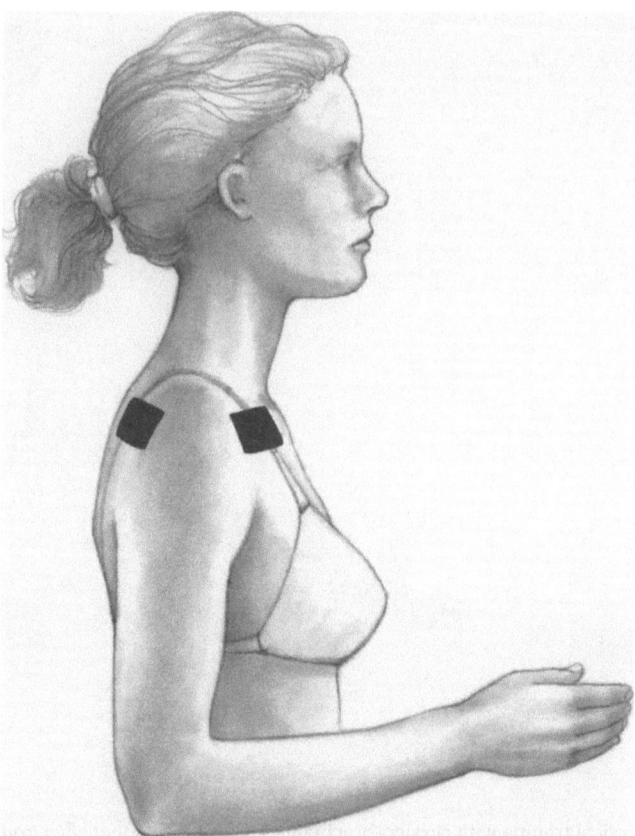

Fig. 4.3. Shoulder dislocation. *Electrode placement sites:* in depression below acromion anterior-ly and in depression below acromion posteriorly. *Recommended mode of stimulation:* high frequency or low-frequency trains, intensity just below pain threshold. *Polarity:* generally of no importance

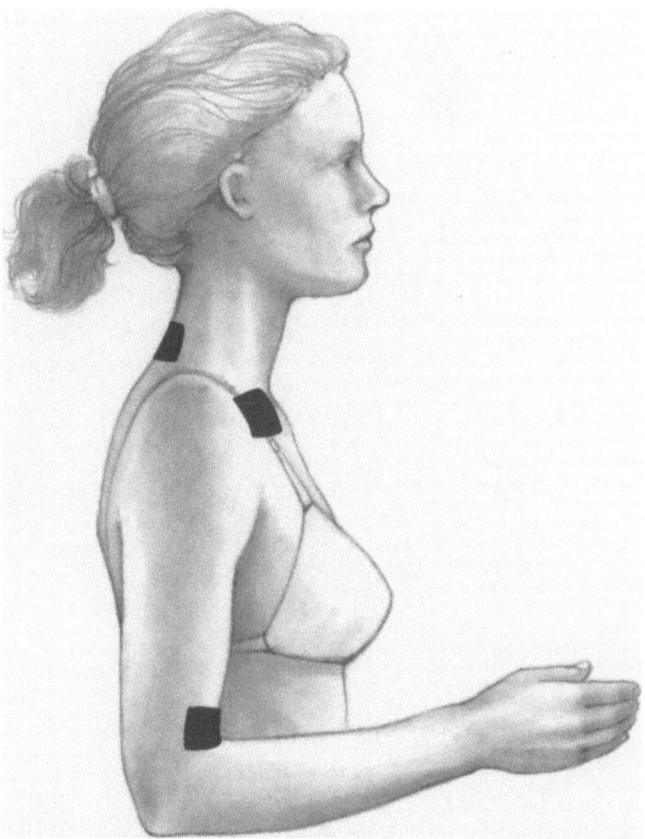

Fig. 4.4. Bicipital tendinitis. *Electrode placement sites:* one pair bilaterally at C5–C7; another pair between first and second ribs just medial to coracoid process and lateral to biceps tendon in antecubital fossa. *Recommended mode of stimulation:* high frequency or low-frequency trains, intensity just below pain threshold. *Polarity:* generally of no importance

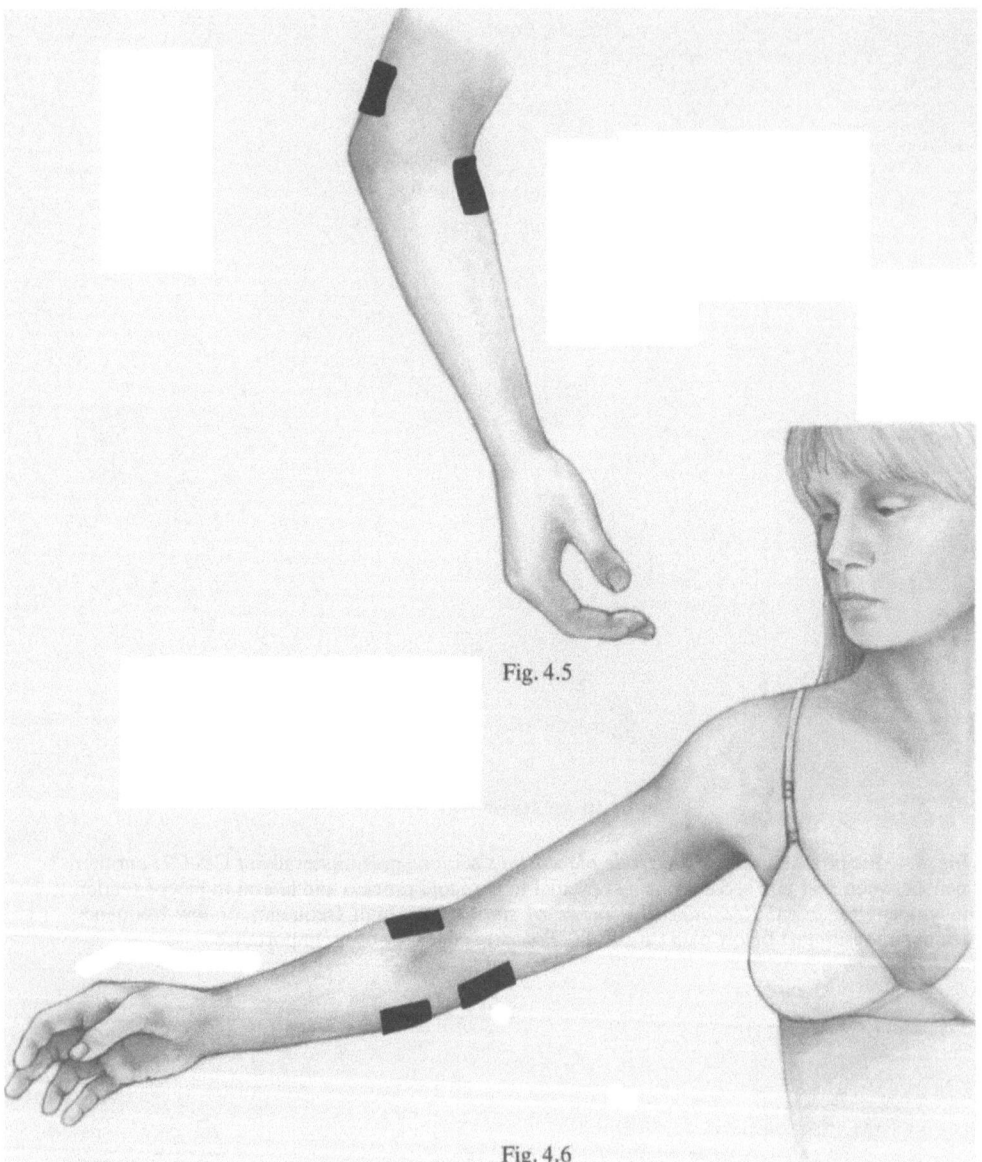

Fig. 4.5

Fig. 4.6

Fig. 4.5. Tennis elbow. *Electrode placement sites:* in depression at end of lateral elbow crease and in depression just above the olecranon. *Recommended mode of stimulation:* high frequency or low-frequency trains, intensity just below pain threshold. *Polarity:* generally of no importance

Fig. 4.6. Post-traumatic olecranon pain. *Electrode placement sites:* one pair in depression just above olecranon and in lateral depression at end of elbow crease; another pair just below groove between olecranon and medial epicondyle and just above medial epicondyle and antecubital fossa, medial to biceps tendon. *Recommended mode of stimulation:* high frequency, intensity just below pain threshold. *Polarity:* generally of no importance

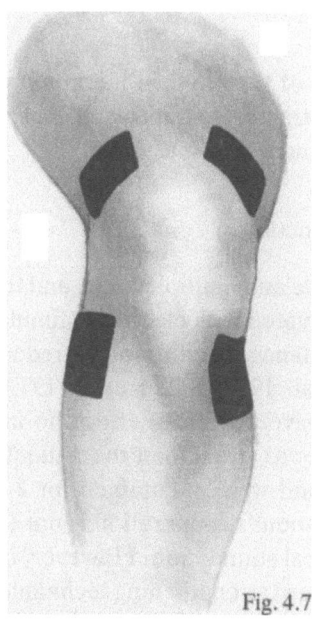

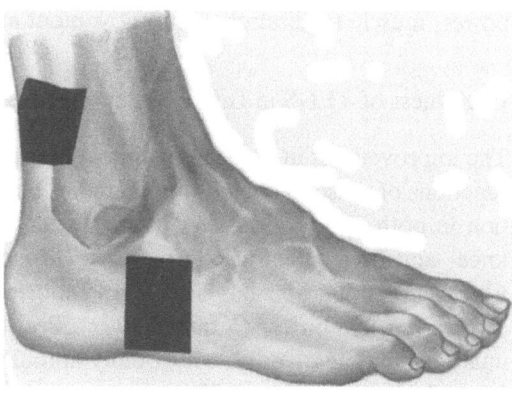

Fig. 4.8

Fig. 4.7

Fig. 4.7. Knee contusion. *Electrode placement sites:* one pair just superior to lateral aspect of patellar base and just below medial condyle of tibia at level of tibial tuberosity; another pair just superior to medial aspect of patellar base and anterior and inferior to fibular head. *Recommended mode of stimulation:* high frequency, intensity just below pain threshold. *Polarity:* generally of no importance

Fig. 4.8. Ankle sprain. *Electrode placement sites:* between lateral malleolus and tendo-achilles at superior aspect of malleolus and just below lateral malleolus. *Recommended mode of stimulation:* high frequency or low-frequency trains, intensity just below pain threshold. *Polarity:* generally of no importance

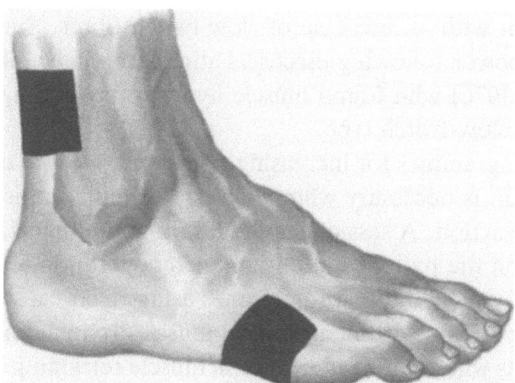

Fig. 4.9. Ankle and lateral foot sprain. *Electrode placement sites:* superior to malleoli on posterior aspect of ankle and proximal to the fourth and fifth metatarsals on the dorsal and plantar surface. *Recommended mode of stimulation:* high frequency, intensity just below pain threshold. *Polarity:* generally of no importance

# Improvement of Muscle Function

Electrical stimulation may be an adjuvant to many of the physical therapy programmes now in use for the management of contractures, improving muscle power, muscle facilitation, limb movement and reduction of spasticity.

## Usefulness of TENS in Improvement of Muscle Function

The improvement in the range of movement of single and multiple joints and the functions of muscles controlling them has been evaluated with electrical stimulation in both upper and lower limbs. It has, for instance, been found to reduce knee- and finger-flexion contractures (Munsat et al. 1974; Baker et al. 1979). Electrical stimulation has also been reported to have beneficial effects in improving muscle power (Kramer 1987). Programmes to strengthen the patient's muscles have involved 4–6 h of daily stimulation and were maintained for 2–6 weeks before significant effects were noted. The patient's cooperation is not essential for a strengthening programme using electrical stimulation. However, involving such cooperation in combination with standard strengthening techniques is more effective. Daily treatment for several short periods of stimulation is preferable to a single long session.

Electrical stimulation programmes have proved particularly effective for patients with orthopaedic problems like arthritis and in those who have been immobilised by casts or splinting. Other good candidates for treatment are patients recovering from upper motor neurone lesions.

Munsat et al. (1974), using electrical stimulation, demonstrated a progressive increase in muscle torque after 2–10 weeks of treatment. Pre- and postprogramme muscle biopsies indicated that the strengthening was due to an increase in fibre diameter. They also reported, in addition to hypertrophy, a change in the fibre type composition, with an increase of slow-twitch fibres. Similar effects of increased muscle power following electrical stimulation have also been noted by Peckham et al. (1976) who found muscle hypertrophy and a fibre composition shift towards the slow-twitch type.

Unlike the programmes for increasing range and strength of muscles, the patient's cooperation is necessary when electrical stimulation is used to facilitate voluntary muscle action. A session should last no more than 15 min and perhaps less, depending on the patient's attention and cooperation and should be given several times a day. Facilitation programmes using electrical stimulation are useful not only for patients with neurological muscle dysfunctions but also for orthopaedic patients who require assistance in muscle retraining following a period of disuse. Neuromuscular facilitation programmes can also be used for patients with partial spinal cord injuries or peripheral nerve lesions. Furthermore, electrical stimulation may be used for sensory facilitation in patients with severe sensory deficits. The proprioceptive, kinesthetic and cutaneous sensibility achieved

by electrical stimulation is sometimes remarkably effective in increasing aware-
ness of a limb or trunk, as reported by many hemiplegic patients (Rancho Los
Amigos Rehabilitation Engineering Center 1987).

Electrical stimulation has been used in several studies as a substitute for an
orthosis in both the upper and lower extremities, and for both long-term functional and short-term therapeutic use. In the lower extremity, its use has ranged,
for instance, from peroneal nerve stimulation to a permanent substitute for an
ankle-foot orthosis.

It has further been demonstrated that electrical stimulation can be used to as-
sist the swing phase of gait in both hemiplegic patients and those with spinal cord
injuries (Stanic et al. 1978; Strojnik et al. 1979). It has been used to maintain stability in the upright position, create momentum and maintain step length (Bajd
et al. 1981). Stimulation of the dorsiflexors during the swing phase of gait in
hemiplegic patients helps in minimising toe drag (Waters et al. 1975). Stimulation of the quadriceps and hip extensors during the neutral phase of gait can enhance stance stability and allow early ambulation for many hemiplegic patients.
Stimulation of the hip abductors during swing can reduce scissoring, while more
intense stimulation provides additional pelvic stability.

Electrical stimulation can also be used in the upper extremity to improve
muscle function. Improved power, for instance in recurrent shoulder dislocations, helps to maintain normal alignment of the shoulder.

Several studies have shown that electrical stimulation may be used in addition to functional training in spasticity and is particularly useful if given immediately before the training session. Different types of electrical stimulation have
been used but three modes predominate. The first is 100-Hz stimulation to the
antagonist of the spastic muscle. This has been shown to decrease tone in the
antagonistic muscle for up to 30 min after the treatment has been discontinued.
Other methods of electrical stimulation are a 3000-Hz frequency stimulation of
the spastic muscle itself or 2-Hz stimulation of cutaneous areas over the spastic
muscle.

Winter (1976) has reported on the use of TENS in six patients with multiple
sclerosis. Electrodes were placed paraspinally between the spinal cord and other
regions of pathology. When paraplegia or paresis was evident electrodes were
placed paravertebrally at the sacrum. Placement was at the posterior aspect of
the ipsilateral trapezius and deltoid when there was upper extremity involvement. Stimulation parameters were of 100 Hz and amplitude settings at the level
of just tolerable discomfort. Results indicated a decrease of painful spasticity
and increased mobility. A 2-year follow-up of 135 cases showed a general overall
improvement with only two regressions.

References

Bajd T, Kralj A, Sega J, Turk R, Benkott T, Strojnik P (1981) Two channel electrical stimulator providing standing of paraplegic patients. Phys Ther 61:526
Baker LL, Yeh C, Wilson D, Waters RL (1979) Electrical stimulation of wrist and fingers for hemiplegic patients. Phys Ther 59:1495
Kramer JF (1987) Effect of electrical stimulation current frequencies on isometric knee extension torque. Phys Ther 67:31
Munsat TL, McNeal DR, Waters RL (1974) Preliminary observations on prolonged stimulation of peripheral nerve in man. Recent advances in myology. Proceedings of the third international congress on muscle disuse, Newcastle upon Tyne, England, p 42
Peckham PH, Mortimer JT, Marsolais EB (1976) Alteration in the force and fatiguleability of skeletal muscle in quadriplegic humans following exercise induced by chronic electrical stimulation. Clin Orthop 114:326
Rancho Los Amigos Rehabilitation Engineering Center (1987) Annual report of progress to the rehabilitation services administration, US Department of Health, Education and Welfare
Stanic U, Acimovic-Janezic R, Gros N, Trnkoczy A, Bajd T, Kljajic M (1978) Multichannel electrical stimulation for correction of hemiplegic gait. Scand J Rehabil Med 10:75
Strojnik P, Kralj A, Ursic I (1979) Programmed six-channel electrical stimulator for complex stimulation of leg muscles during walking. IEEE Trans Biomed Eng 26:112
Waters RL, McNeal DR, Perry J (1975) Experimental correction of foot drop by electrical stimulation of the peroneal nerve. J Bone Joint Surg [Am] 57:1047
Winter A (1976) The use of transcutaneous electrical stimulation (TNS) in the treatment of multiple sclerosis. J Neurosurg Nurs 8:125


Suggested Reading

Bowman BR, Baker LL, Waters RL (1979) Positional feedback and electrical stimulation: an automated treatment for the hemiplegic wrist. Arch Phys Med Rehabil 60:497
Crastam B, Larson E, Previc T (1977) Improvement of gait following functional electrical stimulation. Scand J Rehabil Med 9:7
Currier DP, Lehman J, Lightfoot P (1979) Electrical stimulation in exercise of the quadriceps femoris muscle. Phys Ther 59:1508
Daves R, Gesink JW (1974) Evaluation of electrical stimulation as a treatment for the reduction of spasticity. Bull Prosth Res 22:302
Gracanin F (1972) The role of functional electrical stimulation of extremities in rehabilitation medicine. Europa Mediophysica 8:48
Kralj A, Trnkozy A, Acimovic R (1970) Improvement of locomotion in hemiplegic patients with multichannel electrical stimulation. Proceedings of conference on human locomotor engineering, University of Sussex, Brighton, p 60
Levine L, Knott M, Kabot H (1952) Relaxation of spasticity of electrical stimulation of antagonist muscles. Arch Phys Med Rehabil 33:668
Liberson WT, Holmquest HJ, Scott D (1961) Functional electrotherapy: stimulation of the peroneal nerve synchronized with the swing phase of the gait of hemiplegic patients. Arch Phys Med Rehabil 42:101
Merletti R, Acimovic R, Grobelnik S, Cvilak G (1975) Electrophysiological orthosis for the upper extremity in hemiplegia: feasibility study. Arch Phys Med Rehabil 56:507
Ray CD (1976) Electrical stimulation: new methods for therapy and rehabilitation. Scand J Rehab Med 10:65
Rebersek S, Vodovnik L (1973) Proportionally controlled functional electrical stimulation of hand. Arch Phys Med Rehabil 54:378
Stefancic M, Rebersek S, Merletti R (1976) The therapeutic effect of the Lubljana functional electronic peroneal brace. Europa Medicophysica 12:1
Weinstein MV, Gordon A (1951) Use of faradism in the rehabilitation of hemiplegics. Phys Ther Rev 31:515

# Wound and Fracture Healing

Peripheral arterial insufficiency and leg ulcers due to atherosclerosis or diabetes mellitus is a frequent condition in the elderly. In most patients the symptoms are relatively mild, but in about 10% of the patients it will progress to gangrene. In many of these patients, vascular reconstruction will save the limb, but amputation will be the only alternative in others. Recent studies indicate that TENS and other modes of electrical stimulation may offer alternative methods for treatment of leg ulcers. Some studies also show a positive effect on the healing of fractures.

## Usefulness of TENS in Wound and Fracture Healing

Wolcott et al. (1969) and Gault and Gatens (1976) have studied the effects of low intensity direct current on ischaemic skin ulcers. Wolcott et al. treated 75 ulcers and showed that 40% of the lesions healed completely; all the ulcers except in one patient responded well to treatment. Gault and Gatens treated 100 ulcers; 50% healed by the end of the treatment period. Unfortunately, the control group, which consisted of patients who had bilateral lesions, was small in both studies.

In a study by Lundeberg et al. (1988, in press) the effect of high-frequency TENS on chronic diabetic leg ulcers was assessed in 96 patients. Good results were obtained when the electrodes were applied proximal to the ulcer, within the dermatome. The stimulus intensity was set to four times the perception threshold and stimulation was carried out for at least 2 h twice daily. In 42 patients the wounds healed. The patients in whom the wounds did not heal had reduced skin sensitivity.

Brighton et al. (1979) used constant high intensity direct current stimulation in 168 patients with fractures showing non-union. They found that in 84% the fractures healed. Becker et al. (1977), using low-intensity direct current stimulation in 18 patients with similar fractures, demonstrated a success rate of 72%.

Jorgensen (1977) investigated the effectiveness of pulsating direct current stimulation on healing time in 24 patients with tibial fractures. A group of 33 patients with tibial fractures served as controls. In the treated group the healing time was on average 30% shorter than in the control group ($P < 0.001$). The improved fracture healing in these studies has been attributed to the promoting effect of electrical stimulation on osteogenesis.

## References

Becker RO, Spadaro JA, Marino AA (1977) Clinical experiences with low intensity direct current stimulation of bone growth. Clin Orthop 124:75

Brighton CT, Friedenberg ZB, Black J (1979) Evaluation of the use of constant direct current in the treatment of nonunion. In: Brighton CJ, Black J, Pollack SR (eds) Electrical properties of bone and cartilage. Grune and Stratton, New York, p 519

Gault WR, Gatens PF Jr (1976) Use of low intensity direct current in management of ischemic skin ulcers. Phys Ther 56:265

Jorgensen TE (1977) Electrical stimulation of human fracture healing by means of a slow pulsating, assymetrical direct current. Clin Orthop 124:124

Wolcott LE, Wheeler PC, Hardwicke HM (1969) Accelerated healing of skin ulcers by electrotherapy: preliminary clinical results. South Med J 62:795

## Suggested Reading

Assimacopoulos D (1968) Low intensity negative electric current in the treatment of ulcers of the leg due to chronic venous insufficiency. Am J Surg 15:683

Bassett CAL, Pawluk RJ, Becker RO (1964) Effects of electrical currents on bone in vivo. Nature 204:652

Brighton CT, Friedenberg ZB, Mitchell EI, Booth RE (1977) Treatment of nonunion with constant direct current. Clin Orthop 124:106

Brown M, Gogia PP (1987) Effects of high voltage stimulation on cutaneous wound healing in rabbits. Phys Ther 67:662

Carey LC, Lepley T Jr (1962) Effect of continuous direct electric current on healing wounds. Surg Forum 13:33

Kaada B (1987) Mediators of cutaneous vasodilatation induced by transcutaneous nerve stimulation in humans. In: Sobin A (ed) Neuronal messengers in vascular function. EK Fernström Symposium, 1. Elsevier, Amsterdam

Stefan S, Sansen W, Mulier JC (1976) Experimental study on the electrical impedance of bone and the effect of direct current on the healing of fractures. Clin Orthop 120:264

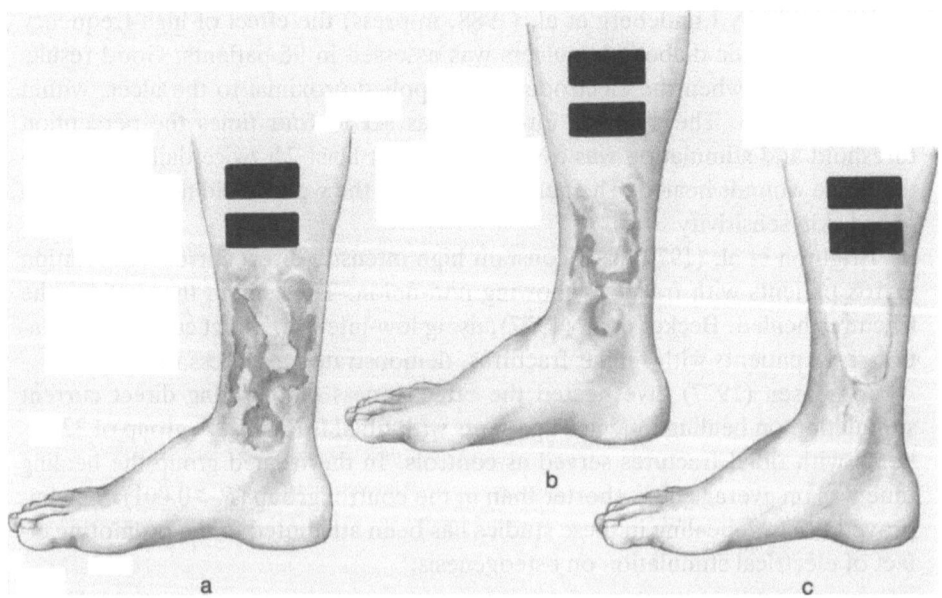

Fig. 4.10. Effect of TENS treatment of chronic leg ulcer in a 72 year old woman. The patient had suffered from the ulcer for 6 years and standard regimen (cleansing, paste bandage, support bandage and exercise) had been of little beneficial effect. a Ulcer at beginning of TENS treatment, b ulcer after 22 days of daily TENS treatment, c ulcer after 46 days of daily TENS treatment. *Electrode placement sites:* proximal to the ulcer, within the dermatomes of the spinal nerves innervating the area of the ulcer. *Recommended mode of stimulation:* high frequency, intensity at pain threshold. *Polarity:* generally of no importance

# Treatment of Venous Stasis

Since the work of Apperly and Cary (1948), many studies have demonstrated the effectiveness of electrical stimulation in the prevention of venous stasis.

## Usefulness of TENS in Treatment and Prevention of Venous Stasis

In 1964 Doran et al. showed a marked reduction in venous stasis using electrical stimulation to the calf musculature during surgery. In a later study by Doran and White (1967), it was found that the risk of post-operative deep venous thrombosis was reduced by electrical stimulation of the calf muscles during surgery. The study was carried out on 200 patients, and each patient served as his own control, as only one leg was stimulated. Comparisons between the stimulated and unstimulated legs showed a statistically significant decrease in the incidence of deep venous thrombosis in the stimulated limb. Similar results have been reported by Browse and Negus (1970).

In plastic and reconstructive surgery, venous stasis often causes tissue necroses and treatment failures. Kjartansson et al. (1988) studied the effects of high-frequency TENS in six patients with surgical flaps after reconstructive plastic surgery. The results show that high-intensity TENS dramatically increases the local blood flow if applied at the base of a flap or proximally within the dermatome. There was no evidence of flap necrosis in any of these patients.

## References

Apperly FL, Cary MK (1948) The control of circulatory stasis by the electrical stimulation of large muscle groups. Am J Med Sci 216:403

Browse NL, Negus D (1970) Prevention of postoperative leg vein thrombosis by electrical muscle stimulation. An evaluation with [125]I-labelled fibrinogen. Br Med J 3:615

Doran FSA, White HM (1967) A demonstration that the risk of postoperative deep venous thrombosis is reduced by stimulating the calf muscles electrically during the operation. Br J Surg 54:686

Doran FSA, Drury M, Sivyer A (1964) A simple way to combat the venous stasis which occurs in the lower limbs during surgical operations. Br J Surg 51:486

Kjartansson J, Lundeberg T, Körlof B (1988) Transcutaneous electrical nerve stimulation (TENS) in ischemic tissue. Plast Reconstr Surg (in press)

## Suggested Reading

Cotton LT (1976) Prevention of postoperative deep venous thrombosis. Br Med J 2:1193

Doran FSA (1976) Prevention of postoperative deep venous thrombosis. Br Med J 2:1193

Doran FSA, White M, Frury M (1970) A clinical trial designed to test the relative value of two simple methods of reducing the risk of venous stasis in the lower limbs during surgical operations, the danger of thrombosis and a subsequent pulmonary embolus, with a survey of the problem. Br J Surg 57:20

Martella J, Cincotti JJ, Springer WP (1954) Prevention of thromboembolic electrical stimulation of the leg muscles. Arch Phys Med Rehabil 35:24

Powley JM, Doran FSA (1973) Galvanic stimulation to prevent deep-vein thrombosis. Lancet I:406

Tichy VL, Zankel HT (1949) Prevention of venous thrombosis and embolism by electrical stimulation of calf muscles. Arch Phys Med Rehabil 30:711

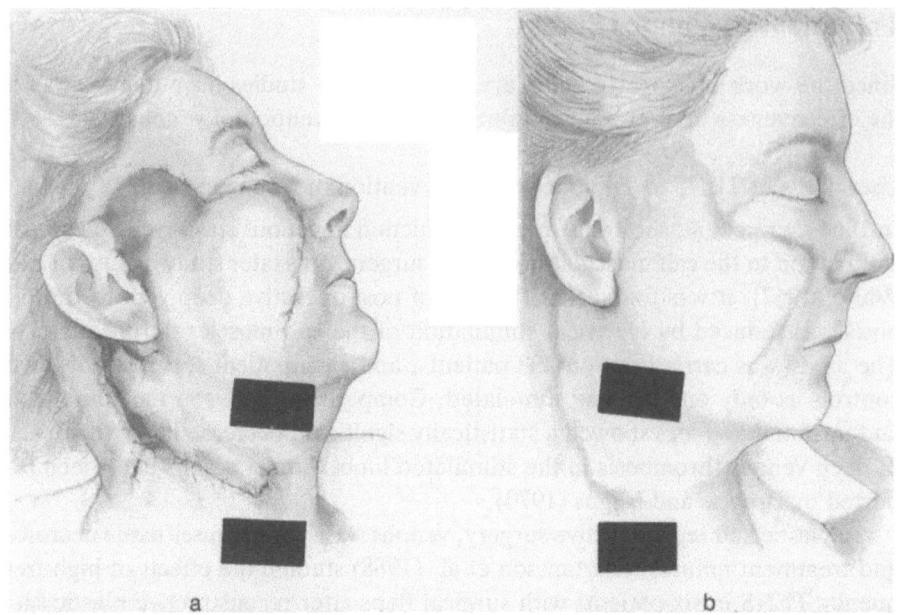

Fig. 4.11. Effect of TENS treatment on venous stasis in a surgical flap in a 60 year old woman operated for a tumor of the right chin. The defect was reconstructed with a transposition flap. 24 h post operatively there was stasis and no capillary refill in the distal part of the flap. a 24 h after surgery and before TENS treatment, b after 3 weeks of daily TENS treatment. *Electrode placement sites:* at the base of the flap, 5 cm apart. *Recommended mode of stimulation:* high frequency, intensity at pain threshold. *Polarity:* generally of no importance

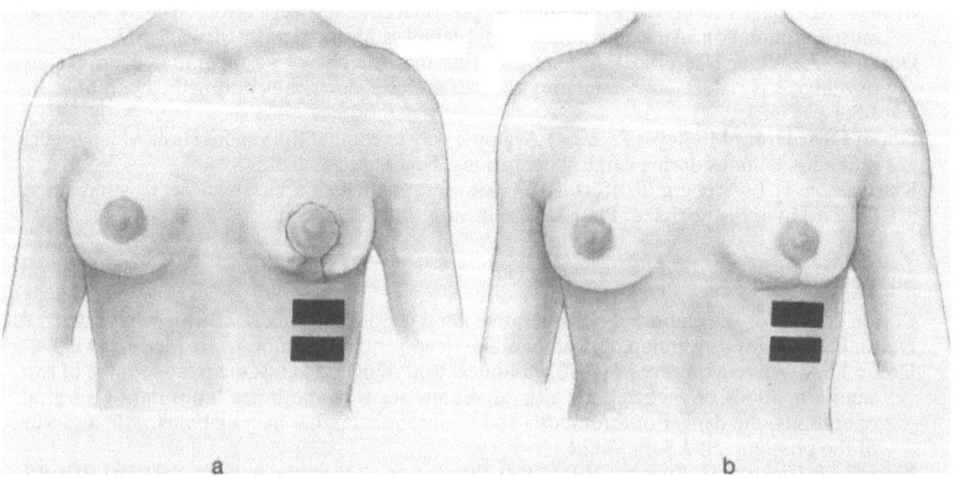

Fig. 4.12. Effect of TENS treatment after reconstructive surgery in a 48 year old woman operated for mammary carcinoma. On the third day after operation there was stasis in the flap and in the mamillae. a 72 h after surgery and before TENS treatment, b 10 days after daily TENS treatment. *Electrode placement sites:* at the base of the flap. *Recommended mode of stimulation:* high frequency, intensity at pain threshold. *Polarity:* generally of no importance

# Pruritus

Pruritus or itching is defined as a sensation which the patient instinctively attempts to relieve by scratching. Itching may accompany a primary skin disease or may be a symptom of systemic disease. First and foremost, the underlying cause of pruritus should be sought and treated. If no skin disease is found, an underlying systemic disorder or drug-related cause should be looked for. If drugs have been ruled out as a cause of itching, one may try tranquillisers, antihistamines or TENS.

## Usefulness of TENS in Pruritus

Fjellner and Hägermark (1978) studied the effects of TENS in 41 patients with itching of diverse aetiology. In a first trial 63% of the patients found that TENS reduced their itching, and 20% reported complete relief. As a rule the effect lasted for many hours, although TENS was given only for 5–30 min. In 15 patients who had suffered from intense pruritus for more than 1 year, TENS was given several times a day for 5 to 47 days. Twelve of these patients were relieved initially, but ultimately only six experienced some benefit from the TENS treatment.

## Reference

Fjellner B, Hägermark Ö (1978) Transcutaneous nerve stimulation and itching. Acta Derm Venered (Stockh) 58:131

## Suggested Reading

Carlsson CA, Augustinsson L-E, Lund S, Roupe G (1975) Electrical transcutaneous nerve stimulation for relief of itch. Experientia 15:191
Gault WR, Gatens PF (1976) Use of low intensity direct current in management of ischemic skin ulcers. Phys Ther 56:265
Kirsch WM, Lewis JA, Simon RH (1975) Experiences with electrical stimulation devices for the control of chronic pain. Med Instrum 9:217

# Subject Index

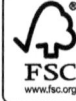

MIX
Papier aus verantwortungsvollen Quellen
Paper from responsible sources
FSC® C105338

If you have any concerns about our products,
you can contact us on
**ProductSafety@springernature.com**

In case Publisher is established outside the EU,
the EU authorized representative is:
**Springer Nature Customer Service Center GmbH**
**Europaplatz 3, 69115 Heidelberg, Germany**

Printed by Libri Plureos GmbH
in Hamburg, Germany